GOOD BRAIN

BAD BRAIN

The Messy Business of Thinking

YOUR BRAIN

Outthink Your Brain and Realize your
Potential

Michaelene Conner
Wellcoach, ACSM, PT, AFAA, Food and Kitchen Coach

MAGIC BULLET PUBLICATIONS, Edition, 2015

3 8 6 3 0 6 7

FIRST EDITION

Designed by Jeffrey W. Doud, MAGIC BULLET PUBLICATIONS, and
CONVERT A BOOK
affliliates of Paragraph and Bmuse.

Library of Congress Cataloging-in-Publication Data
Conner, Michaelene

Good Brain Bad Brain Your Brain

Includes bibliographical references
ISBN: 978-1-939389-70-1

Visit: www.coachconner.com

This book is dedicated to

All the clients I have helped change

All the clients I have yet to meet and

All the individuals who I shall never meet
yet hope to influence through this simple read.

And

To my loving mother Shirley, a health and
Reader's Digest junkie that died from
Alzheimer's. Mom's brain could only take
her so far without mind and body change,
which comes down to a person talking the
language of brain change, practicing the
talk and internalizing substantive
behavioral change.

Contents

A Little Information About Me

Over the years I've worked with and have known amazing individuals from different walks of life. I have always been fascinated by what we think, how we arrive at each thoughtful moment, and the predictability of brain change. My focus has consistently revolved around identifying the "what" and "how" each individual grappled with brain change. I have become the practitioner I am today due to the choices and opportunities given to me. Of course I didn't always feel like they were favorable circumstances but in hindsight realize it forced my brain to go down the roads less traveled. The notion that we reveal the unanswered questions in our lives by the nature of the things we choose to learn and share with others is true for me. My path to mind and body change has felt like a series of psychological boot camp sessions as I follow each person down the path of mental transformation. Wellcoaching has made me the voyeur, the watcher of what it takes to change ones thinking, feeling, and doing. And my clients have afforded me the most valuable tool, knowledge. Whether your dealing with physiological or psychological unwanted habits, I believe *Good Brain, Bad Brain, Your Brain,* will fundamentally influence the way you think about approaching changes in your life. I have seen the writing on the wall and know what lies ahead. Today's technologically managed world is showing signs of mounting complexity and compressed timelines that our brains can't adequately wrap around. Every man, women, and child regardless of their technological agility and need for speed lack the capacity to keep up in this new 24/7 world of continuous information and change. The challenge on the table is not that change is needed or that change is constant but rather the amount of information being assimilated by the brain is creating mental distortion and a dysfunctional view of reality. This mental exaggeration is created with shows like, The New Top Model, reality stars, celebrity chefs and trainers to the rich and famous, the newest voice, endless workout apps, Weight Watchers mobile, and a list of the youngest millionaires or billionaires ever. The magnitude of this new not so normal reality is bouncing around in our brain as the new normal reality we should strive to become. This book will provide insights about the predictability of our behavior, the consistent patterns of brain change, and the strategies that you can use to promote the brain's ability to bounce back from the disruption of change making you better prepared to foster new thinking in this overwhelming digital environment.

I wrote this book because every day I work with individuals that are grasping for a way to explain their circumstances while trying to manage some semblance of success, health and wellness. I hope this read deepens your understanding of how the brain interrupts your life. By learning how the brain thinks you will become proficient in the implementation of SMART brain strategies. My philosophy as a wellcoach has been developed through the practice of teaching others how they can apply what I have learned to successfully implement brain change on the most basic level. This mindset has prompted me to focus on what really matters to people as they encounter life's day-to-day struggles. Everyday I see articles on the Internet and in magazines, brain-memory blogs, advertisements for healthy brain supplements, and endless books on how to help keep your brain intact. Lean in let me share with you a little secret to a healthy brain. It lies in developing a resilient mindset that allows your brain to delay judgement while evaluating assumptions or attitudes you may have about life. This in turn will enhance your capability to influ-

A Little Information About Me

ence your brain's behavior toward unfamiliar information. Then of course there is genetics. Research suggests that more than 40% of societies burden of brain disorders are likely to be genetic. Most of this disease burden arises from complex multi-gene genetics as well as from environmental influences, while the other 60% of successful brain change comes from targeting the right combination of diet, physical and mental activity. These life choices dictate what you do, how you will live your life and what will happen to your mind and body at the end of your life. Your body is like a sailing vessel floating on the high seas, your brain is the captain navigating this complex sea of behavioral brain change. So it makes sense if your brain is working right, you are probably apt to act in a more consciously responsible way that helps you sail through each situation for optimal gains. But when the brain doesn't get the right mixture of sleep, diet, and exercise, there is a higher likelihood you will act impulsively, increasing your chances of poor decisions, health issues, or death. Daniel Amen, MD, author of many neuroscience books has been quoted as saying, "One of the smartest things you can do to increase the length and quality of your life is to optimize the physical functioning of your brain."

If I were asked what do I do for a living, I would have to call myself an urban anthropologist. My digs are client's mindsets, the walls of athletic facilities, and the offices of doctors, physical therapists, psychologists, nutritionists, and RDs. My wellcoaching sessions are like living in a laboratory and have provided me the chance to observe, collaborate, support and analyze the behavior of thousands of groups and individuals as they engage in mind and body transformation. These relationships have given me a rich source of how the mind and body plays out in all kinds of situations. Being able to observe how each individual interrupts and digests information, allows me a deeper understanding of how brain change strategies actually produce results. Everyone nowadays is a specialist. What I've learned is that there is no shortage of snake oil being sold out in the world and there are plenty of opinions being tossed around on the World Wide Web, apps that will change your life, and mind and body programs, all with the promise to bring you positive change. Smoke and mirrors is not my business, I see my role not just that of a wellcoach but as a generalist, which allows me to connect the dots when helping clients address any type of lifestyle change. One theme rings loud and clear; the human reaction to change is the same in everyone but the "how" each individual interrupt change is what matters. This book will give you a glimpse into how your brain reacts to all kinds of circumstance seen and unseen.

Introduction

The Messy Business of Thinking

The brain is the most complex and magnificent organ of the human body represented by a mesh of biology, genetics, and temperament. Composed of 100 billion neurons, each neuron connected to 10 thousand other neurons. Our brains are filled with mystery and revelations processing a constant stream of sensory data. Our brain controls awareness of the environment including voluntary and involuntary movement. It looks forward to life with optimism and fervent aspirations. It can promote success or demise depending on how and what it thinks. Every creative thought, feeling and idea is imagined and developed by our brain. Our brain has the power to provide us with infinite possibilities—retrain the brain and change your life. Grow the brain and reach your potential. *Good Brain Bad Brain Your Brain* is about how your brain thinks and how to grow, understand and reclaim your mental cognizance.

I woke up one day and realized my ability to help people as a wellcoach and physical trainer was very limited. I could only influence the lives of as many people as I had time to train on a daily basis. That is when I decided that I was going to write this book. The problem is that I had only published scholarly articles and knew nothing about writing a book. I decided to approach this endeavor with a beginner's mindset. I found myself receptive, willing yet vulnerable. I came to the realization I had no image to uphold and a desire to help others develop the right mindset, learn more about their strengths while managing their weaknesses and helping to identify the need for new skills so they could be the person they have always desired to be. As an author I have never been influenced by preset rules or so-called acceptable thinking, so each chapter is my way of helping you realize how your brain uses its faculty of reason, allowing you to recognize the gaps in your thinking. This book will not give you all the answers but rather help you ask the right questions. With that information you will be ready to bridge the differences in your thinking with a new mindset. If you're not aware how you live life, the myriad of bad decisions you make over each decade will influence how you age. Your diet and exercise strategy combined with the factors of life stress, lack of sleep, excessive alcohol, legal and illegal drugs, environmental toxins and more influences your brain's stress, strain and health.

Your brain's overall health is connected to your physical wholeness. The way your brain processes information determines your heartiness and happiness. It is the brain's daily decisions that decide the future state of your mind and body. And many times our brains take an anemic approach to health and wellness. To reclaim your brain, you must grow in self-awareness.

To be better at mental transformation on a personal or professional level you need to grow in your knowledge about how the brain talks to you. One-way is to keep a brain awareness diary—daily journaling will give you an opportunity to observe your beliefs and habits and how you think and behave when encountering newness or unfamiliar situations. You can't change your behavior overnight but you can change your thinking now. Many scholars have echoed the mantra that you can't change your thinking by doing the same things the same way.

Yet by learning to change the automatic subconscious thing you do everyday, only then can you change brain paradigms and its cognition to moving your life forward. How do you retrain the brain? How do you change habits? How do you gain new insights and see the opportunities that lie ahead? How does the brain resist change? How do you keep from resisting brain change? Everyone wants to change their life in some way, to improve their circumstance or opportunity for success. I know I do. Yet most people lack the capacity to change their lives remaining static doing the same thing – different day. Stop waiting for your brain to change your unwanted habits because the longer you wait to move forward the greater the probability you will never move forward, drowning in a pool of procrastination. Change readiness comes down to being prepared to want the answer to the questions you wish you had asked. In order to do just that, be aware of the moment and think as if there is no tomorrow but only the now.

I have learned many a lesson on my own path to transformative brain change and the secret to good change decisions is not knowledge but rather understanding how to use that knowledge. Every thought and established pattern of behavior is created by the brain making the process of thinking a messy road, riddled with unforeseen potholes and detours, opportunities as well as dangers, along with an abundance of learning or thoughts that unintentionally deviate from what is correct, right or true. Substantial change is hard to come by because as humans we don't like to think outside our comfort zone. I have learned that our passage though life consists of our brains effort to get the mental maps in our heads to conform to the road on which we walk. Life is about trying to understand where you sit in the world and whether you make a difference. Knowing where you are can be a series of "aha" moments or an ongoing reckoning of trial and corrections. Our mental map represents the constructs in our heads allowing us to avoid encounters and situations that are not in line with our brain's well-established beliefs, behaviors and assumptions of life. Our brain is a life navigation system that is composed of repetitive patterns that determine what we think, say, feel and do. Our brains fear change and unknown circumstances. If you are engaging life in real time you probably don't have all the answers and I am here to tell you that's ok. Our lives are not permanent or perfect and should not be seen as an event but rather a life-learning continuum. Living is about your brain stretching learning, and experiencing itself over and over again. Each day you're thrown into the world, sometimes fully prepared to participate and at other times, confused and caught off guard. Unlike sports specificity there isn't a typical warm-up or as in theater a dress rehearsal. Yet life can be easy to understand if you allow your brain to be a receptor and not a resister of change. Take charge of your brain today. Ask yourself what you would like to change about your life habits, what it would take to make it happen, then plan and prepare to change. The price for brain change is not cheap and the cost is more than we normally anticipate. Yet to acquire significant substantive changes in our thinking we must develop patience and persistence. Deeply rooted shifts in your brain's thinking don't come quickly or easily; there are no quick fixes or short cuts—just practice, time and awareness.

Good Brain Bad Brain Your Brain will help you develop thinking strategies that will assist you in retraining a healthy mindful brain. The most successful brain changes will come from strategically SMART planning. Why? Because to achieve something you desire, there must be a plan, process, preparation, and a practice phase that leads to a repeatable pattern of thought and predictable actions. You and your brain will be asked to invest time and effort to develop a realistic, inspiring, SMART plan that will give you the desired outcome wanted. What is SMART planning? It is a process for predicting a goal based on specifics, able to be measured, tied to action-based behaviors, realistic, and time-lined for successes to occur. Brain change is all about developing a SMART plan that turns your SMART goals into SMART efforts that help your brain to retrain positive patterns of behavior. These well thought through SMART goals are considered SMART because they are customized to your readiness, ability and willingness. For SMART goals to take hold you must start with the end result (the desired state) and a well thought through vision. A compelling vision becomes the framework to create a targeted SMART plan. Your effort must focus on advancing your capabilities (your ability and willingness) within the area you intend to change. This read will give your brain the logistical steps necessary to do just that. Brian Tracy, a motivational speaker and author of *Goals, The Power of Self-Discipline, Focal Point,* and other books has been quoted as saying; "You must ask yourself, what is the most valuable use of my time right now?" That answer will help you shape your brain's thinking and ultimately your action steps towards the new thinking, which will lead to the end result and life improvement.

If you are engaged in living life not merely as a bystander you and your brain will always have too much to juggle as every day is a finite twenty-four hours. Living life to it fullest is about making the most of the time you have, rather than wishing you had more time to accomplish more things. When living life, if we don't take the time to pause and reflect on new information, learning or accomplishments our brain starts to miss significant details in our lives. This book represents three decades of what I have learned about how the brain changes as it relates to the human experience. My investigation into how to retrain the brain is an ongoing exploration that allows me to examine the mental landscape of each client while advancing my own understanding of how the brain changes. In my endeavor to understand human transition I have always considered myself a student first and a wellcoach second. My clients pay for wellcoaching and in return I give them a collaborative partnership in their pursuit of health and wellness. My hope is that *Good Brain Bad Brain Your Brain* will help you understand and manage the mystery surrounding how to change your brain providing you meaningful insights into brain dynamics and useful strategies for life change. In the words from a song written by deceased hip hop legend Tupac Shakur, "I'm not saying I'm going to change the world, but I guarantee that I will spark the brain that will change the world."

1

21st Century Mind Games

The Secrets to Training the Brain

When examining the human brain, the mental capacity required to obtain knowledge of something not yet known before, through observation and study is an amazing intellectual journey. This mental arithmetic represents a process of careful consideration demanding repetition of an action so as to develop or maintain a pattern worth imitating and done without thinking. This systematic pattern then leads to a form of behavior or automatic habit of physical performance as seen in the ranks of tennis, stock car auto racing, or video games. So I guess it was inevitable that scientists would start tinkering with brain stimulation and function to fine tune behaviors and physical performance. When talking about mind and body connections, the science of brain training has taken us to strange and exciting places. In fact, over the past five years Johns Hopkins has done a handful of landmark studies demonstrating that these scientific futurist brain techniques called things like transcranial direct current stimulation (tDCS), which is a non-invasive, painless brain stimulation treatment that uses direct electrical currents to stimulate specific parts of the brain kind of like training specific muscle groups. Several studies suggest it may be a valuable tool for the treatment of neuropsychiatric conditions, which are all emerging depression therapies and actually improve the way a healthy brain can learn and retain motor behaviors. As a professional wellness coach who studies how the brain interacts with the body and how outside stimulants affect the brain, I asked myself why would this be important to mankind? Then it occurred to me that many time the mind gets so lost in solitary thoughts it becomes distracted and unaware of one's ultimate goals and surroundings. In fact the means to support the act of thinking and the processing of that information in a certain way elicits many times an indeterminate amount of mental and physical energy. What scientists are trying to see is if brain stimulation can enhance a persons' ability to perform in todays fast-moving environment, similar to kids playing digital games on their computer, developing strategic thinking, information-gathering, problem solving, visual-spatial skills, adaptation to changing contexts, all this while boosting working memory capacity. As a fore instance, the ordinary iconic game Guitar Hero promotes the development of eye-hand coordination and rhythm skills by allowing its player to utilize an included Gibson SG shaped controller to perform over 30 different songs. These days, individuals from all walks of life are looking to science to enhance mind and body performance. Another example comes from the realm of sport Travis Pastrana, an American motorsports competitor and stunt performer has used the Neurotopia video game for mental training so his brain and body operate automatically as if having done the race or stunt hundreds of times. You may ask yourself why this automatic behavior is important? Because when we expend mental energy we have drawn down on the brain's energy reservoir, which can be thought of as the brain's mental checking account. It seems that when we recover mental energy we fill that reservoir back up by making a deposit into the brain's mental checking account. What this means to human kind is that by manipulating mind and body energy we may be capable of actually managing mental resources or even enhance mental and physical capacity to change a behavior, by directly promoting a positive mental state of resiliency.

RESILIENCY
The Prerequisite to Brain Change

The characteristic of resilience seems to be a prerequisite for change to take hold, and is the single most distinctive element affecting the brain's capacity to engage life. The fact is that having more or less resilience affects the brain's condition when attending to life circumstances. God knows everyone has baggage, yet some people seem to have heavier baggage than others. Think of resilience as a safety valve that helps preserve the brain's mental resources. Becoming a resilient person aids in protecting those mental reserves, which can make a noticeable difference in what will happen in their life. Think of it this way - the more mental resources available, when facing a critical decision or unforeseen circumstance, the faster and more effectively your brain can accept and recover from those disruptions. Developing resilience allows the brain to prosper in today's accelerated and complex environment. When referring to resilience, I am talking about the brain's capacity to absorb mental strain and preserve or improve functionality when encountering adversity or challenging conditions. Daryl Conner, an industrial psychologist defines resilience as ones capacity to absorb high levels of change while displaying minimal dysfunctional behavior. Other researchers have defined resilience as a personal characteristic or sets of traits encompassing sturdiness, resourcefulness and flexible functioning in the face of challenge. As a practicing wellcoach, I've witnessed first hand that all people experience life in accordance to their brain's capacity to take in new information. Some brains seem to thrive on the challenges that adversity sets in motion. These types of brains have been described in the psychological realm as invulnerable even invincible, yet now we refer to this type of brain is simply resilient or stress-resistant. Research has found that the resilient brain has developed the coping skills necessary to counteract risk and respond to challenges that seem to neutralize the impact of adversity and its disruption. This new resilient mindset advances the brain to new levels of adaptation. And it is this ability to adapt that leads to an increased reservoir of resilience or mental energy. So whether we are talking about the resilient, invulnerable or invincible brain, a resilient mindset allows the brain not simply to avoid the most negative outcomes associated with risk, but demonstrate adequate adaptation skills when faced with adversity associated with change. That being said, it is safe to say resilience can be distilled down to the brain's ability to bounce back from experiences of disappointment, frustration or even loss. For instance, when faced with a critical change associated with an unwanted habit, how well we are able to accept then absorb the knowledge about what is needed to change this behavior determines our level of mental disruption, mental distortion, and mental absorption of that information. The speed at which our brains can change that unwanted behavior or moment could be improved only if we understand how to create the most optimal mental and physical environment. And that is where scientific tinkering has been thrown into the mix of brain training.

SCIENCE OF BRAIN CHANGE

Psychological researchers have discovered resilience affects everything we do whether it is learning how to change the body's set point when managing body weight through caloric intake or developing the physical skills needed to adapt to and tolerate exercise intensity during a workout, a serve in tennis, a swing in golf, or a different baseball pitch. When you factor in age, sex, race, or level of wealth, individuals tend not to transition through behavioral change any quicker than their brain's set point to new information allows them. Research has determined the more we try to control our circumstances, the more out of control we start to feel when things don't go the way we expect. If we enable our mind to face danger with courage and self-confidence we lessen the need for control by managing the pressure on our brains mental reserves. This brainy tactic allows us to keep calm while dealing with what we can control. With this increased mental capacity to assimilate change we can rethink our beliefs, behaviors, and assumptions, which indirectly affect our level of control over our situation.

HIDDEN PERCEPTIONS

Perceptions are usually underlying feelings unable to be put into words. The perpetuating cycle of brain change starts with how your brain perceives the change or circumstance. These unconscious hidden perceptions are lying within the brain's neuropathways. The power of the mind, to conceive new ideas, draw inferences and make judgments all comes down to your ability to consciously control years of ingrained patterns of thinking. It works like this, as you consider a new framework for changing a pattern of behavior the degree to which your mental expectations are in line with how you think life "should be" determines how much energy your brain must borrow from your mental reservoir of resilience affecting your assimilation capacity towards change. It's like buying a product or service the "cost" combined with the "want" determine whether the purchase of that product or service will happen. Our ability to look forward to something affects our expectations drawing down on our mental capacity to assimilate change. Anticipation determines whether you feel a sense of control or simply out of control over the change framework challenging your mind's set of ideas, facts, or circumstances that make up life. When dealing with brain change the issue of controlling perception can be a huge mental stumbling block when trying to decide what to change or choose. Look at it this way when you perceive direct control the brain believes it can dictate or shape the outcomes. Conversely indirect control is the brain's ability to anticipate the outcome, which comes down to an exercise in probability. Listen to National Public Radio (NPR), or watch the national and global news it doesn't take long to realize that as a species our need for control is so strong that whole societies focus a tremendous amount of brain power to understand their circumstances so they can manipulate public perception while influencing the events affecting politics, global warming, healthcare, gun rights, abortion rights, gay marriage and religion. The brains of the world collectively stand together in an attempt to surmise, judge, workout, control and make sense of Vladimir Putin and the future of the Ukraine, Israeli's leader signals to a possible Gaza war or Nigeria's kidnappings, climate change, energy conservation, the DNA of Ebola and stem cell research. Whether a case of mental distortion or a case of managing perceptibility, the mental construct is applied to anything that can be apprehended by the brain's ingrained mental patterns and the senses. This sometimes sensible, palpable, tangible or imperceptible mental process connotes the idea is just barely thinkable, visible, audible and so on. The resilient thinker possesses the ability to perceive quickly and easily assimilating information new and unknown at a speed commensurate with the pace of the events taking place in their life. The resilient person approaches the unforeseen information with acceptance, while embracing the challenge. Whole-heartedly knowing the unfolding process is uncomfortable, ambiguous yet able to focus on the desirability and accessibility of the future.

HOW TO RETRAIN THE BRAIN

If you want to change your thinking you've got to question the premise of the ground you walk on. Putting science aside, one strategy is to consistently evaluate your mental activity. When you start to believe or accept an idea as positive or negative, happy or sad, emotionally or intuitively sensitive, learn to recognize and evaluate those pivotal clues by writing it down and talking to yourself about the validity of your thoughts. You do not have to believe everything you think. In fact your brain is a great deceiver. Your mind has a huge imaginary warehouse full of checks and balances, not-so valid facts and unfounded rumors. This simple mental practice of questioning patterns of thinking, behaviors and assumptions can help your brain shift your perspectives, preserving your mental energy, and promoting a change in actions taken. Your brain's level of resilience is systematically bombarded by your past and current existence and environment. There are all kinds of automatic patterns of behavior that determine how each one of us functions. At first sight these firmly established patterns we think are invisible to our brain's inner eye go unnoticed yet influence every step we take. If brain health is an imperative we must learn to expand our mind's capacity to realize what it takes for granted as true while being able to embrace and absorb new information. The pliability of the resilient brain demonstrates its capacity by allowing each individual to sidestep the disruption of unforeseen circumstances in order to rethink the possibilities. The resilient mind is not immune to life's disruption but rather like the beginner at track and field, learning how to take hurdles. Reduced to the simplest terms, the ideal hurdler must basically practice running 100 to 400 meters, while taking what amounts to a long gliding stride over each hurdle. Like the resilient thinker the hurdler will spend as little time in the air as possible getting their feet back on the ground quickly after clearing each hurdle, as they continue running with consistent strides so they can be ready to clear the next obstacle. The mind when confronting life's hurdles tries to do the same thing in order to regain equilibrium and preserve its emotional and psychological health. Everyone at some point has questioned whether he or she should persevere or not. Developing a resilient mindset is the first step to being an elite mental athlete; if you want to be capable of achieving the optimum level of mental performance you must understand and consciously apply the factors that affect your mind's malleability. Retaining the brain's cognitive, emotional, relational or structural mental resources our preserved by applying sufficient flexibility and convertibility to the process of thinking. Resilience is an ordinary adaptive process that doesn't readily occur in all individuals or groups. Yet resilience like becoming a hurdler can be learned. The resilient brain takes 100% responsibility for their actions.

THE BASIC CHARACTERISTICS OF A RESILIENT BRAIN

POSTIVE

The positive thinker tends to be sober about the change decision to be taken. When confronting day-to-day challenge, the positive thinker displays an optimistic view of life acknowledging the complexity while seeing the opportunity. The positive thinker acknowledges that just because a past experience seems to turn out a certain way, that doesn't mean it's a true guide to what's will happen in the future. Yet it is hard for the positive thinker to deny any past experience, which has had a highly emotionally subjective and negative impact.

FOCUSED

The focused thinker lays the foundation for new thinking. The focused thinker delays judgment and identifies needs that connect to a desired outcome. These underlying ideals of future self are the basis from which a compelling vision is developed. The establishment of a meaningful vision in turn supports and justifies **S**pecific, **M**easureable, **A**ction-based, **R**ealistic, and **T**imely **(SMART)** goals. The creation of a compelling vision helps focus new thinking giving an individual the capacity to see what they truly need versus what they have always done.

FLEXIBLE

A flexible thinker can reframe and reconsider a course of thought or action according to the change demands of a given situation. This malleable mindset of the flexible thinker allows that individual to abandon the status quo in order to generate an alternative more pliant plan of action.

STRUCTURED

When exploring innovative solutions the act of constructing, arranging, and organizing one's thinking in the face of adversity is a form of problem solving. The basis for structure enables the individual to invent logical and creative possibilities for real-life-world change. When faced with a variety of information, being mentally capable of narrowing the range of multiple responses becomes key in unlocking the possibilities for the seeds of change to take root. The structured thinker determines the necessary skills and feels motivated to learn and apply those skills in order to succeed.

ACTIVE

The active thinker is both conscious and nimble. It is the kind of conscious cognitive thinking that can make new connections and create new meaning. The active thinker has the capacity to decommission old concepts in order to have internal conversations between the brain's different perspectives.

Active thinking gives the individual an opportunity to anticipate, initiate and create "how" and "what" it thinks of a situation by proactively preparing for adversity rather than responding to it after it has happened. The active thinker understands that change is inevitable and takes a proactive approach by being offensive rather than a defensive student of change.

COMMITTED

Change requires commitment, repetition, and feedback. The committed thinker is open to learning and relearning. This individual possesses the readiness and willingness to move through the transitions and obstacles imbedded in the change process. The capacity to change thinking is enhanced by committed consistent actions connected to a desired outcome. Through constant practice the committed thinker strengthens the required connections between neurons that form through repetition and feedback while weakening the thinking tied to past actions.

The resilient brain is like a high performance sports car built with all the latest technology. This brain has been well crafted for performance with extras like mental flexibility, making it able to take 90-degree shifts in behavior without flipping out. The problem-solver brain has no trouble tolerating the road less travelled or handling the obstacles of a new unknown test track. Here are the rules of the road:

- There is always more than one way to achieve an outcome, if you take the time to think about it.
- A creative and flexible mental attitude will get you everywhere and anywhere in life.
- A compelling vision and smart plan provides the brain the foundation for creative possibilities.
- Success comes with a continuum of trial and corrections leading to enriched thinking.
- Living in the moment and being present is essential for today if you want to be mentally ready for tomorrow.
- The mind's capacity to pause and reflect allows the brain to capture the importance of significant events making those experiences brain changers.
- If you want to grow your brain's potential, sometimes you give up old thinking to grow new thoughts.

2

Brain Strain

Cross Training Your Memory

Today everyone is looking to stay mentally sharp. Yet the sheer volume, momentum, and complexity of our day-to-day lives leave us mentally frayed. To make matters more complex, according to researchers, our brains tend to wander fifty percent of the time, drifting off into thought unrelated to the task at hand – the parent-teacher conference, the groceries that have to be picked up, or what can I get for lunch. The brain could be compared to the Bermuda Triangle in that information pours into our neuro-pathways and seems to just disappear. We are told all through our lives to focus, pay attention; keep our eyes on the ball as we struggle to keep up. The brain is always in thought, controlling what you think, feel, how you learn, remember, move and talk. This doesn't even include the unconscious responsibilities of the brain such as your heartbeat, digestion, and how you manage stress. It is safe to say your brain juggles the demands of life requiring it to be highly organized and focused, personally and professionally.

Then there is our memory of each experience, which shapes everything that our brain does. The act of thinking is the product of careful mental activity channeled by information that we've experienced in the past. The brain's capacity to remember supports our imagination, beliefs, new ideas and the completion of daily activities. The mind holds on to our memories like precious possessions when we file them away in our brain's internal library, ready to be retrieved when needed. Yet many times our memory looks more like a labyrinth. "Memory is nothing more than mental constructions, created in the moment, according to the demands of the present," says Charles Fernyhough, Psychologist. Your memory is the combining of stored sensory and emotional information with formal and schematic descriptions of information about your past and present life experiences, requiring the brain to pull off a seamless collaboration between many different cognitive and neural systems.

WHERE THE BRAIN'S MEMORY RESIDE

If you were to place your finger above the ear and imagine being capable of pushing this area in about two inches, your finger would touch the source of memory. Let's take a tour of the brain. On an initial inspection your brain would be viewed as incredibly compact, weighing just 3 pounds, it accounts for 2 percent of your body weight, and uses approximately 20 percent of our daily calories which comes out to 400 calories if you happen to be on a 2,000 calorie per day diet. The surface of the brain is composed of many folds and grooves, which provide your brain with the additional surface area necessary for storing all of the body's important information. If you scratched the surface to look inside you would notice the brain operating as myriads of little moments. These overlapping moments and sensations now in your cortical cells are decoded in various sensory areas of the cortex, then recombined in the brain's hippocampus forming connections that have never existed before, becoming part of what we refer to as memory. Memory by nature is the mind's faculty of retaining and recalling past experiences through associative mechanisms in the brain—which comes down to the processes of putting information into memory (encoding), maintaining the coded information (storage), and getting the stored information back into consciousness (retrieval). Today the bigger concern is focused on not forgetting which translates into not losing stored information or having difficulty retrieving it.

THE SEQUENCE OF WORKING MEMORY

When discussing memory, the key factor identified by scientists is a special kind of memory they refer to as working memory. The activities associated with forming a working memory entail encoding, activation, rehearsal, and retrieval. Each day your brain comes into contact with people, places, situations, and choices, which we will call stimulus, the neurons in the prefrontal areas of the brain fire continuously in response to the sensations experienced. The reverberation of activity in the brain echoes continuously allowing the brain to make inventive associations between everything you have gone through and felt in the moment combining it with past memories. Working memory is more than the brain's capacity to remember a telephone number long enough to dial it; it is the power to manipulate that information, such as having the ability to multiply, divide, add and subtract, or place that information in different order, sort it from low to high, or having the ability to comprehend a metaphor. There is an important distinction that must be made between that of working memory and mental focus. The brain's working memory has been referred to as a mental workplace that allows you to juggle multiple tasks and retain information while performing the other activities in your life—while mental focus is the ability to sustain, concentrate, associate, and recall a point of origin from which ideas, experiences, and influences emanate. Neuroscientist Antonio Damasio notes that what we memorize of our encounters is not just visual structure but rather a series of multiple consequences of the interaction with our senses, previously acquired memories, emotions and feelings.

The research of Psychologist Nelson Cowan author of *The Development of Memory in Childhood,* depicts working memory as chunks of information stored in memory with contextual markers that point out the situation in which the information is relevant to other experiences. Science labels this as the "restructuring phase" of problem solving causing the relevant information to be mixed together in new ways. In simpler terms neuroscience explains that the human body interacts with objects, people and events while the brain reacts to those interactions.

HOW TO FOCUS ON FOCUSING

The first step towards retraining your brain is becoming aware of each and every moment. The precursor to working memory is the element of attention or lack of it. The environment in which we live and any changes to that environment can drastically affect our power to perform daily tasks effectively while sustaining mental focus. The brain's selective attention is implicit when making those day-to-day decisions or having insights. Home and workplace are booby-trapped with memory's arch foe; the daily unforeseen assurances of "distractions." The extra time on the computer, the last minute meeting, a scheduled client conference or a call from the school that your child is feeling ill and needs picked up ASAP.

The attention process orients the brain to focus on the stimulus of the moment, whether it is your favorite TV show, a speaker at a conference, a fire truck coming down the road or the blinking yellow light at an intersection. Every distraction is well noted by the body's sensory modalities of audio, visual, olfactory, tactile, and gustatory combined with the brain's parietal cortex, which scans the environment around you, analyzing motion, and spatial relationships. This information is then processed, refined, and integrated with the most relevant prior memories experienced moving the thought bytes through the brain's nerve cells forward to the "control nodes" in the prefrontal cortex (PFC), responsible for our actions and responses to information or unknown situation.

The quality of our brain's working memory and focus depends on our ability to handle distractions. These mental intrusions affect the brain's capability to shift attention from one moment to the next. The action of blocking out needless information in a world full of distraction is not an easy task. And it doesn't take much to detour our thoughts. We get home from work, the cell phone chimes and while we are talking to our friend we are putting away the groceries and car keys. Then you realize you can't find your car keys. All your multi-tasking has shifted your mental focus. The evidence surrounding memory retrieval states that it is more or less an automatic process and distractions at the time of encoding, can severely impair the brain's ability to successfully retrieve where you put the car keys. The first exercise towards brain change is becoming more aware focusing the mind is about emptying it of distractions so that one can think clearly. Learn to ask yourself, "What am I doing right now?" If you start thinking about something else that you "must do" that will stop you from focusing on what you were needing to do "right now." Ask yourself how many times have you made a telephone call to someone while thinking about an important aspect of your life only to forget who you called or why you called. We have all had those embarrassing, funny and sometimes frustrating moments. Here's one simple solution for those individuals that have those extraordinary checklists; if it is that important write the "must do" distraction on your daily list to handle later. This will allow your brain to relax giving you the capacity to use all your brainpower for the task at hand. The bottom line is that your working memory should be seen as a limited resource and it's all about how you utilize that resource. Your brain can easily be compared to a muscle having a finite amount of energy or a workout. And when bombarded with too much stimulus, your brain, like any muscle of the body, will experience a power grid overload as in the recent aftermath of Hurricane Sandy.

THE COGNITIVE AND NEUROSCIENTIFIC MECHANISMS OF MEMORY

Neuroscientists have long known that brain cells that fire together wire together. Stronger memories are fundamentally associative, meaning that new information is combined with previously acquired information that are already deeply rooted in our brain's neuropathways. The more emotional or personally connected that person's brain is to the information experienced, the more effective the encoding of the information and its recall. In contrast, if the information is difficult to understand and the person could not draw any parallels between the experiences and couldn't associate the information with already acquired knowledge, the brain probably won't remember may even distort the experience to some degree due the lack of connectivity. These elaborate neuropathways that comprise our working memory step in by recovering stored information combined with patterns of connections and interwoven layers of knowledge that allow us to immediately recognize similarities within situations.

CROSS TRAINING THE BRAIN'S WORKING MEMORY

To enhance mental performance, the working memories of the brain, like any muscle in the body, require constant stimulation through vigorous activity. Researchers describe working memory as the cardiovascular function of the brain. It is believed if you cross train your ability to focus, you can increase your basic cognitive skills that assist you for many other complex tasks. The activity of living life, experiences and learning is the brain's version of the Olympics. Unlike the Olympic athletes who have a limited time to demonstrate their peak performance, the human brain can continue to grow and improve with mental and physical exercise. Researchers now believe that memory has much less to do with inborn genius and more to do with "deliberate practice," a commitment to working at a skill over and over, similar to perfecting your favorite recipe or learning a new exercise.

RECHARGING YOUR BRAIN'S MEMORY

The brain's ability to think, remember and transform itself is the same as a cardiovascular or muscular workout. In order to become proficient, both activities employ intensity, duration, and frequency combined with practice, patience and recovery. When discussing the merit of rest and recovery, research conducted by Barbara Fredrickson, PhD, found participants that integrated mental recovery in the form of meditation display a remarkable positive mental state. After practicing meditation techniques for several weeks, participants in the study showed more mental resources at their disposal than they'd had in the past. They displayed evidence of transformation and growth in mental resources in distinct areas of functionality and psychological resources, becoming more accepting of themselves and seeing their lives as purposeful, enhanced social resources, thus making them feel healthier. It turned out that hitting the mat actually beefed up the brain's ability to handle daily distractions. A Harvard Medical School study headed up by Sara Lazar, Ph.D., reported that adults who practiced about 27 minutes of focused mindful activity a day, including gentle yoga and meditation exercises, had significant increases in gray matter within eight weeks, specifically in the part of the brain that helped to regulate emotions and stress. They believed that those changes reflected an increase in brain activity, which helped the researcher to explain why the benefits of mindfulness continued throughout the day, not just while in class. Scientists have found that individuals who add active recovery to their lives find multiple pathways around life problems and are more resilient and able to rebound from daily stress with positive focus and enhanced performance. Think of your brain as a needle, how you thread that needle and the quality of thread you use makes all the difference when weaving the fabric of neuropathways.

There are numerous lifestyle adversities that stalk your brain's resilient capability and disrupt memory such as:
Stress
Depression
Lack of physical activity
Low blood sugar
Alcohol and drugs
Electrolyte imbalance
Head injuries
Infections
Hardening of the arteries
Insufficient thyroid
Hormone Imbalance
Nutritional deficiencies
Food allergies
Stroke
Food additives
Flavor enhancers
Chemical pesticides
Metal contamination
Unsafe ingredients found in everything from make-up to
    household products
Sleep deprivation

HOW to BEEF UP your MEMORY'S PERFORMANCE

Here are some brain exercises that can enhance your thinking memory. Strategies you can incorporate right now to strengthen neural connections and pathways. Include some of these neurobic exercises into your day-to-day life:

. Get enough quality Zzzzzzz. Sleep is essential to young and old when it comes to cognitive performance and memory. Your brain needs adequate rest and recovery.

. Engaging in any activity that requires your brain to be in problem solving mode like Words with Friends, number puzzles, chess, card and board games will sharpen your thinking memory.

. Tune out distractions and turn down the noise. Be selective with your attention. Focus your attention on things you want to remember.

. After intense periods of mental focus, take a brain break by taking a brief walk or change of scenery.

. Be mindful, focus only on the present moment. The skill of living in the moment provides a means of coping with the challenges of day-to-day living.

. Take a new route to work, stop using GPS

. Learn a new task – a foreign language, Tai Chi, Zumba, golf, tennis, ping pong, paddleball, painting, sculpting or any task that helps develop agility and hand-brain coordination.

. Traveling is a great way to stimulate and strengthen the memory. The early humans gained an evolutionary edge from visiting other cultures by learning and remembering new ways of life.

. Be positive – think positive. Positivity opens your mind up naturally, like that of a water lily, which opens in the rays of sunlight.

. Be socially active. Interact with others regularly.

. Stay focused on the task at hand. Try not to spread your energy among too many things simultaneously.

. Slow down, be present in the moment and mindful of your activity.

. Pay attention to the detail of each moment in your day-to-day life. Find the specialness in the ordinary. Enjoy the unexpected and random thoughts that boost creativity.

. Stay physically active. Walk, run, cycle, swim, or take an aerobic class you have been dying to try out. Physical exercise contributes to a healthier brain and has a direct effect on your muscles and your mind.

. Indirect risk factors that affect the brain, such as depression, stress, hypertension and high cholesterol.

. Eat Healthy – think healthy – be healthy. Minimize your intake of saturated fats and trans fats. Consume only small amounts of olive oil, canola oil, and fatty fish (not fish oil supplements).

3

Frame of Reference [For]

While Dealing with the Slipperiness of Perceptions

Frame of reference (FOR) is a corner stone to mind and body transformation. This mental record of reality represents our past experiences that help shape beliefs, behaviors, ideas, conditions or assumptions that will determine how we perceive, approach, understand and interpret life. Deepak Chopra is quoted as saying "To think is to practice brain chemistry." It was once said we create our own exaggerated worldview. Take a moment to think of all the things you perceive to be true on a daily basis. FOR is the roadmap you use to influence the way you address those daily interactions. And like a roadmap, FOR doesn't show the potholes along the road to changing one's perceptions but simply pulls out specific features such as the turn, split, or shifts on the roadway—similar to being plugged into your car's GPS, which helps you to react to relatively invariable aspects along your journey. Yet, not everyone's mental GPS gets him or her to the same place. The smart brain can listen, value, integrate with, and help others to apply a new perspective.

Frame of reference is an intended or automatic deviation to a variation in thinking. Researchers have long recognized that what we think exists, is not so much a static state as it is a way for the brain to expand and transform information. For example comparing frames of reference within the same classroom, seminar or boardroom can shed an influx of varied perceptions on just about any subject from sports to finance. And when in-group settings a person's capacity to corralling those perceptions and expectations of multiple realities becomes a complex challenge. It is critical to understand the idea that a person's perception of a situation determines whether a shift in thinking will occur. What one person sees as a small wrinkle in the status quo, another may regard as a complete transformation in thinking. As we confront new situations, this sense to understand the moment unfolds due to our brain's ability to recognize familiar patterns. It's like driving home, as soon as you hit a familiar road sign you turn, the brain shifts into auto drive, and further thinking becomes unnecessary. Or you hit a detour and the brain has to recalibrate how to get home. In many ways ones perceptions are the familiar road signs we rely on when engaged in making life's decisions. Our capacity to assess and reframe beliefs, behaviors, or an assumption in life gives us the chance to remake our decisions, making a better choice. Most operating behaviors take place as perceptions of our reality; this mental mirage is the brain's unconscious pair of eyeglasses used to keep our fluctuating thinking in focus. Frame of reference and its relationship to thinking is no more than perceptions shaped by our personal belief systems. And since birth, those belief systems and patterns of thinking have been driven by our brain's experiences, circumstance, context of life, and relationships. The moment another person's viewpoint impinges on our personal FOR the brain processes and interprets all the information surrounding its private perception of this encounter, giving it meaning in terms of probable outcome, emotional values and attitudes. So when managing the thinking that affects differences in perception, one must learn to recognize and appreciate the distinction between there own world and that of those outside their world. As a species we are not very rational. We tend to apply what I call magical thinking to logical circumstances. Are cognitive preferences typically end up steering us in the wrong directions because we aren't trained to think making us vulnerable to new information. If individuals took the time to reassess their perceived choices in a more mindful way they would fulfill their desired potential and improve the health of their mind and body.

Research has found initial impressions create first perceptions, which are near impossible to erase from the human brain and that these first impressions of a person, place or idea becomes our brain's default perception. If we later learn information that contradicts that perception, our brain categorizes it as an exception, rather than using the information to alter the rule. Specifically, we associate the exception with the context of that new information; all other contexts get the "default'"association. Say, for example, your first impression of an individual you meet through friends is negative, yet you end up having an energizing conversation when you run into him or her at the gym and change your mind. In the context of the gym, you'll see the person more positively, but in any other environment whether it be a concert, bar, or restaurant, you'll still be guided by your first impression.

When addressing behavioral change, understanding an individual's singular reality is extremely valuable if you hope to help that individual to reframe or rethink their belief system. These ideas of how our world should operate floats across the wide screen of our minds day-in-day-out. These perceptions represent patterns of interwoven mental activity and become the sum total of what we focus on in any given occurrence. The concepts of perception are portrayed in the Japanese film Rashomon, where four characters give a very different account of the same event. This film reinforces the notion that ones perceptions of reality are both subjective and malleable. It is the truth that each person focuses on different things while experiencing aspects of the same thing. Life's variations are a guarantee because that which seems real from one person's frame of reference is not complete and is not necessarily real from another's person's point of view. Another example of FOR can be found in the world of professional football. Player's rigorously work out, have intense practice and go to work every Sunday to endure a level of physical pain that you or I would find intolerable. The crowd watches in amazement as players incur fractured ribs, concussions, broken limbs, or sprained ankles and yet they get patched up and run back out for the second half. From the FOR of a coach and the player, not going back in to the game would be irresponsible to the team's owner, the team and the fans in the stadium.

Marriage and family therapists have also uncovered similar insight regarding FOR. Therapists discovered it was not uncommon for struggling couples to try to fix their problems by taking a trip, moving into a new home, or adopting a new pet or having a baby. It could be that by doing this, they're trying to create a new context with a new dynamic, one that will stick. Yet it's still the exception, not the rule. So to really change our brain's thinking we need to override and rewrite the default by dismantling or reframing old thinking and replacing it with new thinking. It's certainly possible, but it takes more time and patience than simply trying something new. We must challenge what we know, those deep-seated assumptions we hold about other people, the world and ourselves if we hope to learn how to enact with our thinking. Think of it this way, when we are actively making new mental connections and distinctions, rather than rely on old thinking, we open up and become more alive. And this new injection of mental energy improves are well being and enhances our day-to-day interactions and overall performance.

The above three examples validate the notion every person's belief system has a hidden underlying set of behaviors and assumptions that influence whether the glass is half empty or half full. When it comes to interpreting life, human beings are prone to swaying the truth toward what he or she believes, or wants it to be assigning meaning based on perceptions of a past encounter, situation or event. Things are only good or bad because of the way we decide to look at them—meaning life is 10 percent what you make it and 90 percent how you take it. Generally speaking we don't get what we deserve but what we expect. The mind only sees what the brain is ready to comprehend and can understand. The first step towards readiness is to acknowledge that a shift in lifestyle is necessary.

While there are many theories and extensive research on the preconditions and processes surrounding behavioral change, the most important is the Transtheoretical Model (TTM), developed by Dr. James Prochaska. Most health and wellness coaches rely on the transtheoretical model to help prepare clients for self-changing behavioral shifts ranging from exercise adherence to weight management. The individual can use the TTM as the framework to prepares the their mind to go from "I won't" and "I can't" to the next level of thinking which helps the individual to assess their ability and willingness to suspend judgment, enabling the action of "I might" to "I will." At this stage the individual can mentally agree to accept the new premises on which he or she will act. The final states of behavioral change help the individual think through the actions necessary to shape the "I am" and "I still am" behaviors necessary for transformational change.

Psychological studies have found that people can become so wedded to their particular view of how things should work that they ignore all evidence that suggests that a change in thinking is necessary. For example why do so many of us fail to do what we are supposed to be doing regarding diet and exercise. Our actions prove we understand what to do when purchasing gym memberships, trainers, and nutritional advice yet most of the time we are out of control as seen in the global epidemics of obesity, hypertension, diabetes and heart disease.

I pose the question, is it our biological makeup that inclines us to consume what we should eat, or is it our frame of reference and cultural traditions that need reshaping? Regardless, when making health decisions, an error in perception can have you focusing on the wrong thing, which can definitely mess up your choices about how best to live your life. The coach's task is to help deliver an emotional kick-start to the client's non-conscious mind. But for a change in thinking to take root, you must be willing to reassess your beliefs, behaviors and assumptions of reality. The motivation to exchange old ineffective behaviors with new effective thinking starts with a compelling vision.

Original Source: Adapted from Dr. James Prochaska, *Transtheoretical Model of Behavior Change*. This model is a blueprint for self-change in health behaviors and can be applied in health, fitness, and wellness coaching (Prochaskaetal, 1994).

THE BLUEPRINT TO CHANGE

VISION

The first step to promote a change in thinking is a compelling vision of your desired self. A positive vision gives one a blueprint to work from and the foundation for preparing and planning for effective change. A compelling vision of the future provides one with the motivation, energy and inspiration to start the process of alternative thinking.

PARADOXICAL THINKING

Paradoxical thinking is simply holding two seemingly opposite or mutually exclusive ideas in mind at once. This idea promotes thinking in ways that seem contradictory, unbelievable, or absurd yet in fact may be true allowing the exploration of creative alternatives. You're able to entertain the positive and negative ideas while suspending judgment until you fully look into all aspects of the change strategy. Now we are ready to design a plan.

IMPLEMENTATION

The plan and its details are a critical step towards mapping out newness in thinking. The implementation process is the time to think through things like scheduling, preparation, tracking of performance. The plan needs to identify and investigating the challenges associated with the shift in new thinking. For instance, the barriers or resistance that could surface, competing priorities, lack of time, degree of readiness, willingness, and confidence to move forward. Clearly defined action steps are next.

ACTION

This is the time for ritualized skill building. Action is all about the "doing" part of the change strategy. Remind yourself that this is a commitment to the mastery of a new behavior or skills. To reinforce your motivation and confidence, it is important to experience manageable successes that lead to extrinsic (external) rewards, and an intrinsic (internal) value for the new behaviors. One way to transpose the hurdles of new thinking would be the intense conscious rehearsal of required actions and a strategy to reinforce each behavioral goal.

GOAL

Pick one goal that you really want to achieve. Now figure out what it would take to achieve that goal. Effective goals are **S**pecific, **M**easurable, **A**ction-based, **R**ealistic, and **T**ime-lined (SMART GOALS). **SMART***goals raise your awareness of how this change in thinking challenges your thoughts and emotions. This thinking/feeling work will help you in the development of realistic first steps in moving forward.

*Doran, G.T. (1981). *There's a S.M.A.R.T. way to write management's goals and objectives. Management Review*, Volume 70, Issue 11(AMA FORUM), pp. 35-36.

Ask yourself "do I possess the readiness, ability, and willingness to achieve this goal?" If you're not ready, ask yourself what would it take to get ready. If you feel you lack ability, then search out training and if it is a willingness issue take a look at your belief system, negative thought patterns and perceptions that perpetuated resistance in the form of mental barriers to the desired outcome.

RESULTS

Gloria E. Anzaldua author of *Borderlands/La Frontera: The New Mestiza* was quoted as saying, "Like all people, we perceive the version of reality that our culture communicates. Like others having or living in more than one culture, we get multiple, often opposing messages. The coming together of two self-consistent but habitually incomparable frames of reference causes "un choque," a cultural collision."

In other words, you can't change the old brain behavior without new information and new associations. Einstein once said, "Problems cannot be solved by the same level of thinking that created them." The successful adaptation of new behaviors and the absolute confidence that it can be sustained is an amazing feeling. One's ability to absorb new information requires commitment, patience, allotted time and a diligent continuous effort.

DESIRED STATE OF ME

Lasting change expands our sense of self, which allows us to get closer to becoming our best self. Our new self is buried under an old belief system riddled with extra-physical and emotional baggage. Newness is your source of inspiration and motivation.

A primary cause so few individuals achieve what they really want is that they lack the capacity (ability and willingness) to reassess their fundamental beliefs. Or perhaps people find themselves in a more strange and lonely place in their thoughts, thinking they might not be able to share with other people to the degree they'd like to because it's beyond other people's perceptions. Our Frame of Reference consists of an effort to get the maps in our heads to conform to the ground on which we walk. FOR determines our expectations, which influence what we perceive and how we process all knowledge about specific subjects or situation. The information and learning we've acquired since birth drives our unwavering firmness of character and actions. This self-perpetuating cycle is often a major source of our biases to newness and the resistance we unconsciously harbor when the map doesn't agree with the ground we walk. This unconscious automatic thinking creates and reinforces our concept of reality shaping our social space, conversations and rules of engagement. These beliefs create the mental narratives we use when we talk about art, music, religion, politics, sexuality, and more importantly the plots of our favorite

TV shows. Positive or negative, it seems that our reality and morality is no more than the brain's record of multiple consequences of past interaction. And on a daily basis we act on these multiple faded memories using past knowledge of comparable situations, similar to the one we perceive to be experiencing.

Shifts in one's thinking occur through conversation that encourages that person to entertain new ideas and changes in behavior. This requires the person to do more listening, more inquiring, and more reflection. Substantive brain changes is a collaborative and co-creative partnership between old and new thinking. Many times we are actually held back in our lives when we worry too much about how others perceive us. Questioning one's FOR challenges what they believe to be true and how it affects their life's story. We tend to view our FOR as a "measurement device" that helps us elicit information that will give us answers. Who we are, what we think and feel not to mention what we do represents the sum total of what we believe to be true effecting every decision and action taken. Anthony Robbins said, "Beliefs have the power to create and the power to destroy." The human species has been given the ability to take any experience and create a meaning that disempowers them or one that can literally save their lives.

CHANGE YOUR THINKING CHANGE YOUR BRAIN
Here are some re-framing techniques we can us to instantly move us to a place of consciousness.

1
AWARENESS
The fork in the road is not the end of the road unless you refuse to take the turn. Mental flexibility opens your mind to a new narrative. When rethinking your life, consider the way you're looking at a problem, situation or issue might very well be part of the problem itself. By paying attention to your thoughts and feelings you can increase your level of awareness and invest in

what you want and where you want to go. Life is inherently neutral and you and your brain assign the meaning.

2
UNTANGLE YOUR MIND

Get to the heart of what's bothering you or what you'd like to change. Question the premise, rather than accept what seems to be true. After all, don't revolutionary and innovative solutions occur outside the box? Doesn't breaking established thinking lead to newness. Liberate yourself from ineffective self-defeating behavior then get out of your way. Choose to break your rules in order to change the future.

3
CONTROL

The perceived degrees of personal control over decisions play a key role in determining whether the event will lead to success. Know when to slow down your thinking and apply the brakes. Ask yourself, "Do I inhibit my impulses and do what is right? Or do I do what I want in the moment?" Resist the temptation to waste time or engage in any activity that is worthless or harmful. Being successful is about inhibiting ineffective actions while implementing beneficial actions.

4
BRAINSTORM

When you reject change you become the architect of decay. Admit new possibilities. Evaluate the pros and cons associated with your perception of reality. What are the costs and benefits of not changing your way of thinking? Be aware of thoughts and feelings associated with your decision to change. You're not judging or blaming yourself; you're simply exploring opportunities.

5
BE PATIENT AND TAKE YOUR TIME

Fostering growth by not forcing it. Quality time doesn't happen because you set time aside, but rather by playful thinking and curiosity. Find your own creative answer. Notice when you're feeling stuck, walk away, and come back to the problem later with a fresh perspective. You'll be amazed how your mind comes up with solutions if you give yourself time. Acknowledge that not everything you believe is black and white. Be honest and courageous with yourself and look at your present state thinking through new eyes.

Evaluate your perceptions from a place of respect. Mindfulness is the non-judgmental awareness of what is happening in the present moment. We tend to walk around on automatic pilot most of the time, become fully aware of where you are and what you are trying accomplish.

6
CHALLENGE

Realize that what works for one may not work for all. To promote new thinking, challenge your perception of reality from multiple perspectives. New thinking helps to decontextualize those ingrained beliefs, slowly loosening their power over your mind. But when you challenge your new thinking using your old beliefs, behaviors and assumptions, you simply sabotage brain change. Allow yourself to be mentally flexible by accepting the challenge and preparing to navigate the inevitable sea of change transition.

7
RECOGNIZE

Recognize that people behave in the way that they think their life should be. Listen to the metaphors you use verses the metaphors used by others. Thinking begins with perception. Change the image – change the meaning. Our perceptions of reality speaks to life's narrative about ourselves, others and life around us. This narrative begins at birth and is equal to truth. Whether the learned perception is true or false makes little difference your brain. It is important to recognize that the perceptions we have heard, learned, and believe to be true came from someone else's perception not our own, and their perceptions came from some misguided individual who also has been given this information from yet another well-meaning individual.

8
HOPE

Most of the time we're not consciously aware of our feelings which are actively running in the background of our mind and occupying our attentions and intentions. Our degree of awareness claims our influence and how we see the world. When changes in perception are introduced into our lives, reality begins to shift. For every human being, the concept of hope is the one idea that intuitively keeps us on track, feeds positive feelings and inspires an empowering mindset.

9
POSITIVE

Changing your thinking, leads to creativity, imagination, and better discussions with yourself and others. Practicing a positive way of perceiving one's reality, and taking the steps to change those practices, results in a change of thinking and behaviors. It's your belief that creates your current reality and assigning new meaning to those thoughts can change your current and future effect on reality. Your perception of reality can be good, bad, positive or negative, upset or calm. Every cell in your body is affected by your thinking. Negative thinking is like dumping pollution into your lifescape and destroying your mind and body with toxic thought.

4

The Mind of Resistance

When Thinking Won't Shift

Resistance to change reflects the way the mind thinks about an event, tightly held assumptions and values or current state of mental conditioning. One of the most valuable tenants when managing resistance is to understand the nature of perception and the role it plays when shifting ones point of view. Resistance to change is not a black or white issue but rather a landscape of grey, resulting from a number of complex reactions and inter-actions experienced over time, coded and decoded into logical predictable patterns within our brain's neuropathways. How we perceive anything in life plays an integral part in whether we accept or oppose a particular shift in the status quo. Resistance to new thinking refers to the overt and covert actions we take to block out or discount new information that is inconsistent with our perceived view of reality. Unfortunately most times we don't have direct control or influence over what happens to us yet we do possess the capacity to influence how we interpret what hap-pens to us and how we react to what has happened. Richard Lazarus (March 3, 1922 – November 24, 2002) was a prominent psychologist who believed that emotions are extracted from our appraisals of events that cause reactions. Lazarus's appraisal the-ory focused on the notion that emotions result from one's inter-pretations and explanations of their circumstances. Our thoughts about unforeseen or challenging conditions are key factors in whether we confront, resist or implement a coping strategy. Your mind's capacity to allow shifts of thinking sends the message of being less judgmental and less pessimistic or more positive. This state of mind gives the brain a chance to deal with the taunting sometimes intentionally provocative conditions we come up against. Change and resistance to change is routine in today's global society whether talking politics, technology, health care, religion, or marriage. And no matter what you do you can't stop life from changing any more than you can control the weather. If you fail to question "what," "how," and "why" you resist change, you've become part of the problem left behind and unable to adapt to your future needs. If you're not part of the solution, you are part of the problem and clearly defined by what you won't do rather than what you are open to try. Life is neither positive nor negative but rather full of trials and corrections. Your mental attitude towards change determines your emotional quotient (EQ) and your emotional state determines your level of resistance.

Our species can be divided into two categories, those individuals who view life's challenges as opportunities – opportunity oriented individuals are the "glass is half full" type O personalities that see the complexity and potential in each situation as a source of growth and learning. Then there are the danger–type D oriented individuals who see the "glass as half empty" against a backdrop of pitfalls and problems; just the thought of change immobilizes their actions making them scared and complacent. Individuals who resist change are likely to find themselves mentally lost or worse, boxed in and passing through life with an inability to cope with their resistant mind, which can lead to stress and psychological problems.

Even if life seems negative there is often a positive viewpoint "if" you take the time to question the ground you walk on. Only you have the power to shift the mind of resistance, allowing you to grow from unforeseen or uncomfortable circumstances. When dealing with unexpected events or glitches in daily life, the brain can be compared to reading a mystery novel, what may lie ahead is not yet known and next steps are unpredictable. Our brains tend to look for ways to create certainty instead of shifting perspectives by pulling up established beliefs, automatic behaviors and unquestioned assumptions. The brain's demand for homeostasis is the minds natural need towards equilibrium and away from the demands of a change in thinking. The brain is hypervigilant to identify any shift in our environment because it prefers to revisit what is familiar. Even when confronted with a negative behavior the mind can make the case that nothing needs to change. Due to the element of uncertainty; humans are inclined to side step undesirable or seemingly threatening situations due to their preference for familiarity. For example, friends in abusive situations, a spouse with destructive patterns of behavior, or addictions, sometimes it is just easier to live with a problem when you know the cycle of behavior. Trying to cope with uncertainty becomes a bigger issue than the problem.

RESHAPING THE MIND OF RESISTANCE

When thrown into a pool of change the brain initiates the "resistance trap" by questioning your established frames of reference (your view of reality) and invalidating incoming new information. This state of uncertainty means the brain must manage emotions, information or circumstance now open to more than one interpretation like a political speech filled with ambiguities or a binding agreement created by a law firm. The management of multiple interpretations pushes the mind to generate new thinking that allows the brain to process and use information to create a fresh operating framework. Coping with resistance is to discover practical information and skills or attitudes and actions you can use in the face of a changing environment. Resistance to change can mean different things to different people. How we interrupt these differences defines yet again our level of resilience when confronted with mental disruption. Everyone experiences life change, disruption and resistance to those life changes. We can leverage our brain's capacity towards a shift in thinking by understanding how certain factors affect our ability to bounce back from new or unforeseen situations. A common thread in humanity is that everyone on the planet moves through life at a unique psychological pace that allows him or her to make sense of his or her day-to-day encounters. Our brain's capacity for change requires us to recognize "how" the mind transitions through the reshaping and transition process. And in order for the brain to transition past and current thinking there must be a marked departure from previous practices while setting the stage for new expectations that will allow success in the existing unprecedented environment. Just the idea of initiating new thinking starts to question the long-standing beliefs and patterns of behavior. Our reluctance to believe or accept is used to maintain old practices and defy new rituals that affect the brain's neuropathways through the process called "self-directed neuroplasticity." The notion "practice makes perfect" allows the brain's neurons to fire and connect through neuroplasticity. The more we practice any skill from parallel parking to playing Black Jack or using a new software package resistance starts to fades and the easier it becomes to navigate a fresh environment. However in today's contemporary complex time deprived society are brain is now faced with psychosocial stressors, for which, resistant thinking must access our higher, thinking and problem solving area of our brain. Reshaping the mind of resistance take patience, time and the practice of new patterns of behavior. Our resistance to change can be overcome through learning and the continuous practice of new thinking. There is the belief that neurons that fire together wire together, the brain's thinking is not set in stone in that we possess the ability to reshape our thinking and in doing so make our brains more resistant to the stress associated with change. Yet it is naive to think changing years of deeply rooted beliefs and behavioral practices can be flipped like a light switch—it will take readiness, willingness, commitment and consistent unwavering practice to make a dent in reshaping the mind. While the mind of resistance is reluctant to change when new ideas, information and behaviors are being examined, the acceptance and establishment of new thinking starts to develop a track record for success within the brain's neuropathways. These positive experiences reinforce and promote the brain to buy into the next change effort making it that much easier. According to many neuroscientists it can take six to nine months to create new automatic behavior. For example it takes high performance athletes days, months, and years to perfect their skill and consistent performance. Changing the mind of resistance starts with small wins. Even before your brain really believes the shift in thinking is suited to one's end or purpose, it is beneficial to start behaving as if it is a favorable idea indicative of future success and morally sound. Cognitive psychologists suggest our behavior informs our attitudes and help shape the characteristics of happiness and wellbeing. Don't expect that the resistant mind of change will accept transitions without a full-fledged battle. But if you spend all your mental energy in defending your brains strongly held beliefs instead of moving forward, you're damaging your future opportunities.

HOW CAN YOU IMPROVE THE MIND OF RESISTANCE

Why can't people just change for the better? Well you don't know what you know till you question the mind of resistance. Neuroscience is learning a lot about the "why" factor when we resist change in the face of a more promising future. Neuroscientists have found that resistance is as normal and involuntary as falling in love. Yikes! Meaning we are a sophisticated species able to create complicated circumstances which requires painful thinking and many times consequences. The brain can be divided into the "primitive fast-thinking monkey brain," which quickly assesses incoming information, compares that input with stored associations and routines. Even the most sophisticated thinkers rely on the hidden monkey brain for their day-to-day perceptions and decisions. Then there is a "slow-thinking human part of the brain," a central processing unit which tries to understand the facts of the current situation, recognizing, reasoning through decisions, mindful awareness and learning. The use of the human part of our brain is agonizingly hard work. We rely heavily on this slow-thinking area of our brain to help give us clear direction or to make sense of our environment and systematically test new strategies. This type of brain activity is energy intensive and causes the pain associated with mind and body change. The human brain must embrace trial and correction, heartbreak, delayed gratification and challenge after challenge in order to overcome the barriers that the hidden monkey brain presents. These events may seem black and white yet they all require mental adjustments in the way we conduct our lives and make decisions. These new conditions cause resistance even when they're seemingly positive. Improving your reaction to change rather than lose your mind simply requires mental adaptation in outlook, shifting your view of reality by decommissioning past beliefs and being receptive to new thinking. When dealing with a changing environment keep in mind that there is a continuum between black and white, opportunity and danger, or positive and negative outcome. In every life episode the brain has a tendency to control and define how our lives should play out and whenever something occurs in our personal soap opera that is inconsistent with our understanding of reality, we brush up against the mind of resistance. The brain's capacity to withstand the not yet experienced future is not easily codified good or bad. Psychological factors such as level of resilience; perceptions, beliefs, behaviors and assumptions are all part of the resistance equation. When we experience life in a specific way day in and day out, we develop core belief system, which make up our view of how life is supposed to be. So in order to change the mind of resistance a person must acknowledge and modify their environment, situation or physical and mental condition lending to the circumstance that defied their existing view of reality. Because our brain operates on autopilot, our mind can be pretty irrational when identifying changes and discrepancies in our environment.

When dealing with change resistance new information can

be really bothersome to our thinking process. The mind of resistance seeks out like-minded people that reinforce our beliefs and discount all information that is in sharp opposition or following no predictable pattern with our view of reality. And when like-minded groups agree, it's even easier to write off the opinions of others in the face of established verifiable facts, discounting conflicting incongruous information as bias to what the mind knows as true. Essentially the disruption caused by discrepant knowledge about a specific subject or situation is met with a sea of resistance. We resist because our brains hate loss. When we invest time and energy, days and months or years in specific patterns of thinking and behavior we cling to our beliefs that much harder because we refuse to lose the time and effort applied to a specific situation. For instance we resist ending a work or love relationship because we don't want to accept the consequences of an unknown reality.

The brain struggles with "what" went wrong, "how" could this have been different, and "why" me. Instead we view resistance as an inevitable part of life. The brain is more like a software upgrade. As your reality evolves with the introduction of new information, unforeseen circumstances, demands, and compressed timeframes, the brain becomes painfully clear that the old operating system doesn't work anymore. At this point the mind of resistance starts to take over, wanting control and predictability. Whether the series of events are seen as positive or negative the mind's psychological neuro patterns decipher the sequence of events experienced during the change process. It is critical to keep in mind there is no black or white but rather a continuum of grey. Shifting gears, like installing a software update never comes without emotional stress, complications or consequences. Yet with consistent practice your brain will loosen its grip on resistance allowing the mind to embrace uncertainty.

5

The Brain's Need for Patience and Time

When Thinking Won't Shift

As the saying goes, practice makes perfect, and you can acquire patience the more you and your brain repeat an action so as to learn, change or maintain a habitual way of behaving. Malcolm Gladwell staff writer for The New York Times and author of *Outliers, Tipping Point,* and *Blink* was quoted as saying, "Practice isn't the thing you do once you're good. It's the thing you do that makes you good." As you can imagine, patience is very important in reaching any goal, nurturing a relationship, acquiring expert knowledge or becoming an amazing cook because it requires practice and study, skill building and the application of knowledge resulting from experiences of practice over long periods of time. The implementation of patience requires time because in most instances reaching one's goals takes much longer than expected. In today's fast paced world patience has become a time critical emotion that fuels the energy or anxiety needed for perseverance and proficiency. In my health and wellness practice I am amazed at individuals who enter the change process with their eyes half open unconsciously committing to a behavioral shift or weight loss program only to give up not realizing substantive shifts in behavior takes time and patience. And many times these highly committed individuals set goals only to give up before they start to see results due the lack of patience and realistic timelines. Your brain needs to embrace the mindset "good things take time," even in the face of unforeseen setbacks and tough situations. Any sports professional will tell you even if there seems to be little change or improvement; no matter how you feel, do the practice every day. This idea applies to anything from managing your diet to pitching baseball. In the context of lifestyle change the lack of patience is why people quit before the seeds of success can take root. Patience is the capacity to tolerate time, delay, setbacks, and frustration. If you want to change something you must submit to becoming patient and decide to be relentless in your commitment to self-discipline. Patience is the one thing many people don't develop because the world has become an instant environment. The mental attitude of being patient doesn't come easily to most of us in this techno world of disposable brief hits of information. The patient brain allows the necessary time to determine what is needed to overcome obstacles. The fleeting concept of time is an essential component when the brain needs to develop and implement new strategies. Other factors that influence the brain's ability to initiate or to switch off the emotions of patience are those of self-control, heredity, culture, environment and life experiences. Malcolm Gladwell author of Outliers: The Story of Success point to the fact, researchers have settled on what they believe is the actual amount of time required to develop implicit expertise about 10,000 hours of practice which reinforce the need for your brain to be patient. Surely you have heard someone say, "Wait, be patient, the storm will pass." In today's unpredictable global environment patience is short lived while the need for speed to keep up in this new world is continuous, accelerated, complex and sometimes downright chaotic. The brain's ability to willingly suppress restlessness, life's little detours and disruptions, or an annoyance when confronted with delay seems absurd in technological terms. The characteristics of bearing provocation, misfortune, or pain without complaint, loss of temper, irritation, or the like is seriously not going to happen. In our mentally hyped-up, faster-is-better culture, try standing in the endless lines at your supermarket. What you witness is people looking at their watches, heavy sighs, and cell phone conversations and then eventually over the loud speaker, the manager announces, "all cashiers report to your registers." Or have you ever driven on the freeway, behind someone who was actually driving the speed limit continuously as people pass them at an accelerated pace? Even authors like Martin E. P. Seligman, Ph.D. and Barbara L. Fredrickson, Ph.D. the mavens of happiness and positivity fail to mention the concept of patience in their many books of happiness, positivity and learning—so tell me again, why do I need it? Then, I asked myself; why amid so much technological efficiency is there still no patience and persistent time-poverty? It seems a turbocharged life is still the ultimate trophy on the mantelpiece. As if status is determined by one not having to wait for any wants, needs or desires.

In today's transformative society it is a mark of being hugely important when you're brain thinks it can't wait and believes you simply don't have the time or patience to tolerate the moment. I know I have moaned a time or two to the tune that, "I'm so busy, that my life is a blur, and I haven't got time to do anything" as I have my own private pity party. It is my belief that patience remains in existence to make our brains less vulnerable to the attacks of stupidity, anger, and annoyance in the face of delayed satisfaction. Wolfram Schultz, Professor of Neuroscience at Cambridge discovered that patience is controlled by a group of neurotransmitters giving our brains the ability to detect signals in the environment, which allow an increased probability of reward within a specific time frame. And our mental time frame is determined by the duration of effort required based on past experiences. Yet scientists found the brain doesn't really compute anything, it simply senses neurological patterns. So I asked myself why are we so impatient? In evolutionary psychology and cognition neuroscience, patience is studied and categorized as a decision-making problem, involving a short-term choice or a long-term choice. Think of patience as a pool of water that evaporates over time. Once the pool has dried up, you're less likely to keep your cool when faced with a similar situation. A great example of the brain's battle with patience and time frames can be witnessed when you're on a weight loss diet. Not buying or eating your favorite foods is a short-term challenge. But not buying or eating those same foods ever again becomes a long-term hell. The practice of slowing down and becoming patient requires the brain to remain focused, alert and actively engaged in the change process, which comes down to the brain making a realistic assessment of the time needed to achieve a desired outcome. Oh, and by the way one's sex has no preference as men and women are equally susceptible to faster-than-thou one-upmanship. Over decades the adult brain has unconsciously crafted a "microwave generation" – where younger brains have lost the ability and willingness to wait for anything. Everything must be made-to-order within minutes! Including relationships, financial endeavors and personal gain. As a society we've created generation after generation of excited, energetic and consuming young brains. The lack of patience has become a trait of "being American" not to mention the global landscape of how different cultural groups live life and do business. The notion of I needed it yesterday has been and continues to be imbedded in each new generation's thinking, their manners, communication style, perceptions, and relationships. On a personal and professional note I've learned that the important things in life usually require more patience than we expected and cost more time and money than we anticipated.

Edgar Cayce, an American psychic, was the first to allege there were three planes that govern the earth: time, space and patience. His idea was if you managed your efforts and stress levels you could enhance patience, changing your relationship to time and space. The concept indicates that the health of our mind and bodies could be a direct manifestation of our state of mind. Duh! Just pick up any health journal, magazine, or newspaper, and we can read or Google a version of Cayce's message in everywhere being written by today's contemporary health minded authors. Here is the secret; patience has a lot to do with time and your stress level, making patience more like money. We even talk about being "time-rich," or more often, "time-poor." So, I wager to say if you're time poor, you're likely successful and impatient. The answer to how patient we will allow ourselves to be lies in how we think about time itself. It seems the American culture is more prone than others cultures to race against the clock. Patience does not run parallel to slow motion and too much patience seems to overlap with the anti-globalization crusade. Then, there are those who believe that turbo-capitalism without a measure of patience offers a one-way ticket to burnout. A Google search on patience will turn up scores of sermons railing against the demon speed. Patience requires simply a pause now and then, allowing one to assess where they are going, how quickly they wish to get there and more importantly, why. It is a brain imperative to question the need for speed. Because allowing the brain to wallow in patience can expose the beauty of experiences or reveal what a situation really has to offer. Life is filled with its ups and downs. The problem seems to be that that our brains simple want the ups without the downs.

Our society obsesses over fast Internet speed, losing 20 pounds in two weeks, making your first million in your 20's, immediate exercise results, and getting everything you need and want now! Not now but right now… or better yet yesterday. Actually, two days ago! Patience may seem like an under-utilized moment, but these seemingly flat periods within each day, become quiet moments paused for our brain to reflect on past life experiences, encounters and situations, which provides the brain a glimpse of what may lie ahead. Life cannot be an ongoing crescendo; there must be some dynamic contrast. Without patience the brain tends to rush the moment, miss the learning, see less, feel less, and hear less. Hurrying the present moment allows us to perform all the daily vital tasks of life on a lesser level. Ironically, the buzzword multitasking and the concept of patience are an unlikely relationship. Multitasking involves rushing to get things done usually at the expense of patience. The "must have it now" haut monde mindset goes against a quality existence. With patience comes greater forethought and opportunity, by helping one's brain to sort out the things that actually matter most from the things that matter least. And time is what a lifetime is made of; everything in life requires the calculation of time, yet many live on borrowed time taking it for granted. You have heard the expression "time is money". Money problems can be corrected but time is simply gone. In other words, how you spend your time is more important than how you spend your money.

David Gray, a social business consultant with Dachis Group explains that management of change takes time. Gray believes you can't help individuals, groups, and organizations introduce new technology and related processes, mergers and acquisitions without some degree of patience. Daryl R. Conner, author of Managing at the Speed of Change and a global thought leader in the field of change management has spent his entire career demystifying the techniques and patterns surrounding the time and patience it takes to change organizations, leaders, and the implementation of change within corporate cultures. Gray and Conner agree that change and its management is not a once-in-a-while thing and should be viewed not as an event with a beginning-middle-end but rather a continuum state forcing the hand of patience. Conner goes one step further by saying, "Prepare yourself for constantly escalating disruption, and expect more than you can anticipate." Conner's research points to the fact that the volume, momentum, and complexity of change initiatives versus the time and patience required for our brain to actually change the landscape of a life or organization has accelerated beyond our capacity to predict specific events. And to make matters more difficult, the turbulence of world events is spreading on a global scale making event predictability less and less reliable and patience a luxury. A current example is the Middle East uprising or the handling of the Ebola virus. Analysts are describing the turbulence surrounding these world-changing events as a steady state of existence similar to living in a house with the lights on 24/7. A contemporary instance of how our brains may lack patience can be illustrated through our levels of consumption—the idea of instant gratification is pervasive. Case in point, as a nation we are brainwashed to believe we live in a world where healthy diets, regular exercise, and the use of supplements and creams combined with plastic surgery can change the future and roll back time. On a daily basis our brains hear about the beautiful people and their beautiful friends, in their fantastic cars, living in their dream home. Somewhere along the rocky road of happiness our minds have become impatient, wanting quick fixes to all our woes. With the click of a mouse, technology tends to shortcut any hope of allowing patience to take hold. Why be patient? Why not move at the speed of light or at least the speed of sound, which is four times slower than a speeding bullet. When reflecting on the lack of patience it seems we tend to lose our patience when we are multitasking or when we're on a tight schedule, as if expecting the day to pass within only a few short minutes. Impatience tends to creep into the day slowly, in an unapparent manner making your brain feel a sense of anxiety. A common illusion entertained by those searching for lifestyle change is that it can be applied like a formula or taken like a pill. Instead of allowing our brains to become impatient, we should be reflective thinkers uncovering the thought patterns that are positive, unhealthy or destructive to your next pressing decision. Patience allows your brain to explore and learn about changes you seek yet patience can only be cultivated and nurtured over time, not days, minutes or seconds. It should be obvious by now that any process directed at substantive behavioral shift, are those generated gradually through well-established patterns of new thinking. These new practices require the brain's effort to permit time to pass, insights to be explored, giving us the ability to try new approaches! If you really want to succeed in this life and not merely live, you must practice patience by being consistent day in and day out. You will never change your brain or your life until you change your relationship with time.

If we really want to participate in and enjoy a meaningful existence and not just attend this experience called "your life", then you may need to buy into the truth of slowing down your thinking, taking a moment to decipher each instance in time rather than simply respond to an urge in the future. The brain's role of time, patience, and reflection is really that flicker of consciousness; without space between musical notes there can't be a beautiful melody or harmony, right? So how does one develop patience? By remembering that patience is a mental skill to be mastered by your brain. And, as cliché as it may sound, life is not a race but rather a journey full of experiences to be enjoyed and remembered after lessons have been learned, applied and used as a springboard to life satisfaction. Here are some simple strategies to becoming more self-aware:

Ask yourself, 'why am I in such a hurry?' Try to think through why you are in such a hurry. You can then think logically and decide whether your impatience is warranted. Not focusing on what matters most in life tends to fuel impatience. Target the triggers that influence you to lose your sense of patience. What are the circumstances surrounding your feelings of impatience? Then look for patterns of behavior that lend to your feeling of impatience.

Just like a food log brings awareness to a dieter, journaling your patience or impatience can be an eye opener. Committing your thoughts to paper can lead to a better understanding of yourself and thought process. Get in touch with that "I need it now" feeling. This newfound awareness will help you identify alternative strategies.

Change your attitude about your life's circumstances. Assess your perception of a situation. Ask yourself, what is real, valid, or relevant. Without understanding the powerful effect of your viewpoint, it becomes virtually impossible to appreciate why your reaction leads to impatient behavior in the first place.

If you can't do anything about your circumstances, move on. Don't waste emotional energy with situations you can't control.

You are never a victim of situations holding few consequences like waiting in the line at your grocery store or post office. In fact, be prepared to wait in line with a book or tablet in hand or check emails on your phone.

Take time to experience the happier moments in life. Think about the times you've felt completely moved? The last time you were truly happy about an outcome. They were probably instances where your extra time paid off; good things may not always follow in the wake of those who are patient, yet most good things come with the passage of time and are worthwhile?

Practice makes patient. Like any brain exercise, new thinking creates new neuro-pathways to new behavior. Gradually the old reactions and urges weaken while the new behaviors take root allowing you to gradually develop the strength and tolerance to remain patient when encountering the most trying and enduring situations. Some forms of human existence take time and cannot be rushed. For instance, when recovering from a having a baby, surgery, mending a broken limb or losing 250 pounds, the law of patience points to the notion that if you work hard at something, in most instances you have to apply patience and time to get exactly what you want. The secret to patience is simple planning for more than you anticipated because sometimes "shit just happens." Reframe and reassess all the twists and turns in life and think of them as an introduction to unfamiliar and unforeseen opportunities.

Be still. In the words of Eckhart Tolle, a widely recognized spiritual teacher of our time, best known for his writing on "The Power of Now," sit quietly and think about absolutely nothing. Learn about YOU! Yes, so you're missing the occasional ping on your phone, Instagram or Tweet, and you're starting to feel impatient after a few minutes, yet by practicing this mental form of time out, you will essentially teach your brain to slow down and focus. Try not responding to your technological devices on demand. Abandoning your cell phone, digital devices, tablet or laptop for 30 minutes to an hour shouldn't be a loathsome task to fulfill. In fact, this kind of quiet should be welcomed. Your new mantra, "Life doesn't run on a perfect schedule" and "Technology doesn't control my life, I control technology."

Stop holding yourself and others to an unattainable expectation. Life would be great if we didn't get flat tires, appointments didn't run late, computers didn't crash, global melt downs came to a halt, and human's didn't make human mistakes, but that is never going to stop.

Now you are ready to answer the question, why be patient? It is easy to see that once you possess the ability to change your thinking, you will start to change your attitude regarding the slowness of people and situations. As your brain applies patience you will start to become aware of a newfound tolerance for unexpected disruptions and minor offsets. These glitches in time should be embraced as common practice. You will start to notice how you have a higher tolerance towards the disruption of any trial or tribulation. The strategies you and your thinking create will help new patient behaviors take root on a landscape full of impatience. As a strategy if you were in a doctor's office and the only thing you could focus on is the your time being wasted, I imagine your capacity for patience would fall by the side of the road. So exercise your patience and bring something you can work on to keep your brain occupied. Research has shown that individuals who stop to think about their lack of patience tend to become more aware, calmer, and accepting. Nobody is perfect and if you develop a patient brain you may actually gain new insights about yourself. Patience is the foundation for a healthy mind and body, reducing stress levels while improving quality of life and longevity. But the biggest payoff is that patience can make you and your brain happier.

6

Techno Stress

Technology: Is it Enriching Your Reality or Replacing it?

Yes, there is such a stressor. We are no longer hitchhikers on the information highway. We live in a world of connectivity and it is growing every day byte by byte. Stressors arrive on your doorstep daily in various forms: chemical, physical, emotional, neurological, environmental, and now technological. When talking about technostress we are referring to the brain's reliance on technological devices, which induces a state of near-constant stimulation, from being perpetually "plugged in." Technostress simply put is technology-induced pressure. The idea of saving time is joined at the hip with the high value we place on planning for the future.

A hundred years ago our greatest minds started to visualize a more efficient world where advances in technology would make life highly productive, consistent, and profitable. In return these technological marvels were supposed to give us more time for friends, family and ourselves. For instance, the technological invention we call the printing press didn't subtract an economic value from society; rather it engendered an explosion of value that benefitted all mankind. Our brains are invaded on all fronts from computers, incoming E-mail, voice mail, chiming cell phones, TV, online games, DVDs, laptops, tablets, iPod Touch, iPad, The Kindle Reader, The Sleep Number and the list keeps getting bigger and better. Technological stress has become a national epidemic.

The sheer speed of the technological experience produces an extreme future that impoverishes our present moments. What ever happened to the concept of "savoring" life? Isn't that why all these devices came about in the first place?

We are like frogs in a simmering pot of technological change and we can't even identify how this connectivity has affected our brain's stress levels. The first inkling that there may be a problem came in 1984 when Craig Brod, author of Technostress identified the human cost of the computer revolution and the emerging problem as a modern day disease of adaptation caused by an inability to cope with the new computer technologies in a healthy manner. The symptoms of technostress during this period ranged from irritability, headaches, nightmares, and resistance to learning about the computer or an outright rejection of the technology layered with pressure in the work place to accept and utilize these new techno devices. Today's information intense IT environment lends to the feeling of diminished human intelligence, less capable in comparison to most machines. The question is how are the relationships and activities that our brains are connecting to online changing what it means to be human and how we think about life? To value technological and virtual reality over our humanity is a choice that will collide with over a hundred thousand years of the brain's biological wisdom, amputating our senses and crippling our ability to feel. Granted we are no longer able to live in this world without being involved with some form of technology.

But aren't we all super human carrying a myriad of mobile devices complete with Internet access? Technology may have a brain and store your info in the cloud but behavioral economist Richard Thaler refers to the human brain as a slow, erratic central processing unit making it almost impossible to handle more than several things at the same time. The end result is our minds create the illusion that we can multi-task. But isn't that why we have technological devices? For instance, every one at some point has caught his or herself cooking dinner while talking or texting a friend on the smartphone, doing a load of laundry and watching their favorite TV show. I've done it, and you've done it. Technology has given our mind the false perception of "multitasking." Even though technology enables our brains to maintain the illusion that we can do many things at the same time, the brain becomes overloaded and stressed out trying to keep up. During techno overload, your brain flips your body's switches in an attempt to absorb large amounts of information in order to act on a decision or the processing of information, to acquire knowledge, to achieve higher levels of understanding, and for maximizing performance through learning. Your brain relies on a kind of mental accounting but it has limited processing abilities. We are not like a computer with the capability of storing or minimizing information. When involved in techno interactions, interruptions from sources such as smartphones and computers, there is a break in concentration, mental focus and continuity. According to researchers, with each interruption it takes approximately 25 minutes to get back to work.

A 2005 study sponsored by Hewlett-Packard found the average worker lost 10 IQ points when interrupted by ringing telephones and incoming e-mails, which they equated with missing an entire night of sleep. These techno timesavers turned out to be the very devices that we are told will make our lives more efficient and easier; yet promote unexpected mental and physical consequences. "This cortical flaw has been exacerbated by modernity", says Jonah Lehrer, author of *How We Decide*. He points to the notion that we live in a culture that's awash in information; it's the age of Google, Twitter, Facebook, cable news, Wikipedia, and LinkedIn. Because of this instant second to second processing of information bytes, our mind gets anxious whenever we are cut off from all this knowledge, as if it is impossible to live, work or make decisions without being plugged in 24/7. With all this technological advancement comes an invoice. The hidden cost lies in the human brain; it wasn't designed to deal with such a surfeit of data. And within all this technological opportunity is the danger that we are constantly exceeding the capacity of our brainpower. Jonah Lehrer makes the analogy that it is like trying to run a new computer program on an old machine; the antique microchips try to keep up, but eventually they fizzle out.

The media consistently reminds us that "connectivity" is the tidal wave of the future and many times it feels like a tsunami. Technology has increased the availability of information exchange and the speed at which that information can be acquired, giving our society a digital camera, instant gratification mindset much like the Polaroid of years past. In fact the world has become interconnected to the point of mass hysteria and mental distraction. You can't tell the gossip and rumor mill from the validated facts when hearing it online or in the news. The pure volume of information being consumed in your techno diet produces information fatigue syndrome. What scares me is that technology has changed our perception of time and has altered our internal clock to fast forward for information acquisitions, which in turn leads to unrealistic expectations. As in the movie CLICK starring Adam Sandler, a harried workaholic meets Christopher Walken and gets his hand on a magical remote that he uses to fast forward, bypassing life's distractions; he mutes conversations, skips unpleasant situations and really lives an empty existence. In the end Sandler realizes how he has basically missed out on life, family experiences, valuable learning, health and wellness. But Herbert Simon, Nobel Prize winner and late professor at Carnegie Mellon University said it best: "A wealth of information creates a poverty of attention." Technology has saddled our ability to think with blinders and has left us with a diminished understanding for what it takes to be world class; distorting our thinking and dulling our value for human excellence through the process of "intellectualizing and digitizing" monumental human achievements. This growing mindset has radically altered the way we build our personal and professional lives and how we interact with others.

Technology is here to stay, a permanent brick in the wall of our society—it is still in its infancy and we are just learning its effects on mind and bodies. These devices will only grow in use, and with it the technostress we experience. Let's not substitute our day to day reality with the virtual reality of cyberspace which can only clash with decades of biological wisdom, amputate our senses, hamper our feelings and perpetuate stress. As a group of people united in a relationship and common purpose, I will leave you with this thought bite—as a society we need to balance our humanology with our need for technology. If we don't focus on the amount of technology we consume, we will start to normalize the cascading abnormal behaviors taking root in this new growing techno scape.

TECHNO STRESS
How You Catch it

Technostress is just another modern day brain addiction. The symptoms associated with this disease I referred to as "techno-centered syndrome" range from irritability to a high degree of factual online research and thinking, poor focus, limited access to emotions, an insistence on efficiency while displaying lack of empathy for others.

In 1984, Craig Brod coined the phenomenon in his book *Technostress* which identified the techno trend as promoting breaks in concentration, feelings of being overwhelmed, and a high degree of anxiety. The tools we use shape our minds and the human species is being shaped by these technological interactions. As a self-aware creature we are impressionable; subject to strong mental or emotional responses and able to receive and respond to the external stimuli of technological stress; the state of being constantly stimulated or perpetually "plugged in." I see it everyday, people glued to a cell phone or texting while driving or kids consumed with computer games or television. This growing mindset has radically altered the way we build our personal and professional lives and how we interact with others. For instance, instead of confronting the "how", we react to techno stressors that cause mental and physical sickness and prefer to focus on "what" we can fix with medications for sleep deprivation, alertness, mood, indigestion, relaxation, and sex. We don't regard technostress as a potential problem.

Once you have the disease it affects the brain giving people a diminished ability to accurately estimate how long a task really takes to complete. This leads to constantly overestimating performance standards and timelines in the workplace and dampens one's ability to manage their time effectively. This newfound perception of efficiencies is a false reality often leading to neglecting extra time for outside activities. Our sped up mental framework becomes a "time warp" increasing levels of frustration, anxiety and criticism of self, others and the workplace.

Even the human genes and memes are evolving at different rates. Genes refer to the makeup of all living things. Then there are the memes, which refer to ideas, messages, and opinions that are shared and modified within the human species. Given memes can replicate and mutate thousands of times faster than genes thanks to the internet, humanity has become pressured, stressed by changing ideas well before our cells have a chance to adapt, creating mental disconnects and high levels of dysfunction. What we play with reveals what kind of species we will become.

Sadly technology increases time spent in sedentary work habits. Sitting before a computer screen or accessing other technological equipment for long periods of time increases mental labor, which in turn consumes a tremendous amount of energy, leading to a deep, emotionally based fatigue that is quite different from physical fatigue. At the end of the day the inexorable advances associated with this "time saving" technology meant to help us stay more connected serve instead to keep us from ever fully disengaging.

Technological devices have overridden the brain's natural rhythms that once defined the human species and now blurring life's boundaries. Technostress is just like any other addiction; you become an excessive-compulsive addict interacting with technology. The stress hormones adrenaline, noradrenaline and cortisol fuel arousal and create the need, the rush and the high of being connected. When we decide to put our mind and body on the back burner, we are eventually going to receive an invoice in the form of necessary healing. This technological addiction has produced a population that is fragmented, lacking purpose, depressed, and filling doctor's offices with an array of aliments, without intimate connections, and isolated from community support.

Another perspective was brought to the forefront in an article from Wired magazine, titled "Why the future doesn't need us." Bill Joy, CEO of Sun Microsystems rants that the enormous computing power combined with the manipulative advances of physical sciences and the new, deep understanding in genetics open up the opportunity to completely redesign the world, for better or for worse. Joy predicts that the emerging technologies are likely to profoundly alter humanity and even life on earth. He leaves us with the parting thought that as a species we are far from understanding how genetic patterns turn into organisms, yet we are well along in changing those patterns and thereby changing science from a way of understanding how nature works into a tool for changing what humanity will become.

TECHNOSTRESS
How you Cure it

Stress is categorized in various forms, chemical, physical, emotional, neurological, and environmental. Technostress interacts with all other forms of stress to create a synergistic effect $(1+1=6)$; for example combining alcohol and painkillers. The two sided blade seems to indicate that technology lets us accomplish so much more and in today's fast paced, complex, demanding, and sometimes turbulent world, people take on too much and end up feeling overwhelmed with no end to the work load. To disengage from technology has become a thing of the past and nearly impossible. Connectivity is the tidal wave of the future and in many ways it is penetrating our world like global warming.

One of the most pressing problems associated with technostress is that our brains don't get to unwind or recover. There is this continual, unrelieved build up of stress on a chemical level, which in turn eventually contributes to a behavioral and/or physical problem. Technostress hits us on an emotional level and emotions control our hormones through biochemical changes in the brain. Whether these techno stressors are labeled good or bad, stress depletes the mind and body hindering its ability to perform efficiently. When technostress reaches extremely high levels, stress becomes a concern. That's because of the effect of the stress hormone cortisol. When you operate on full throttle your glands become exhausted, and you end up with low levels of cortisol and no back up to increase the hormone.

SYMPTOMS
Symptoms of technological stressors on the brain are:
. Feelings of memory loss, forgetting what you started to do or why you walked into a particular room
. Impatient with self and others
. A lessened ability to relax or slow down
. Anxiety over having lost access to your smartphone, tablets, TV or other types of techno equipment
. Headaches, stomach discomfort, back pain, ulcers, and irritable bowel syndrome (IBS)
. Difficulty falling asleep or staying asleep
. Continuously checking your e-mail, voicemail, surfing the web, and other types of techno equipment, and not turning it off for the night

THE CURE
Managing Technostress

Ethel Roskies, author of *Stress Management: a new approach to treatment* makes the point that stress has become the fashionable disease of today and the treatment for stress is a popular and profitable activity. The commodity called stress has created the need for stress management methods. To manage the high-tech addiction of overload, we must go to the place it originates, the brain. To help the brain retain cognitive fitness, we must look at factors that affect the brain:

. Glucose (sugar) and H2O (water) – Low levels of glucose (hypoglycemia) and dehydration significantly affects the functioning of the brain. Eating complex carbohydrates, fresh fruit and vegetables is a great way to replenish glucose and not feel run-down. The slow release of glucose from complex carbs keeps the brains energy level consistent with less dramatic spikes representing a healthier choice then that of simple carbohydrates like fruit juice, candy or sweet treats which break down immediately causing the body to have dramatic spikes.

. Hydration—Keep your brain hydrated, about 80% of your brain is actually water, and the rest of it is taken up by both physical and biochemical structures. Your brain uses about 25% of the oxygen and sugar that your body circulates for nutritional needs.

. Rest - Recovery, downtime and sleep. Studies show that optimal amounts of sleep range from 7 to 8 hours per night for men and 6 to 7 hours for women. Ignoring sleep is like stalling to pay your credit card, if you don't things are only going to get worse. Sleep and rest are a necessity not a luxury.

. Time Management - Give yourself more time to do everything by building a margin for error. Schedule time to take care of specific daily tasks.

. Time Out - Set regular "Time-Out" periods or simply go outside and take a break or meditate.

. Self Care - Meditate, Stretch, and Exercise. Get out of the office or home and do some deep breathing.

. Eye Strain - Take a short vision break every 30-minutes

. Focus on the Moment - Limit multitasking and practice being present.

. Boundaries – Make clear distinctions between work times and free times. Limit the times of the day when you check emails, cell phone, play games, watch TV or access other technological devices. Use technology to create and publicize your boundaries. Educate and contract realistic timelines with others.

. Prioritize – Ask yourself what is of primary importance in your life. Think about what refreshes you and deliberately plan to fit that activity into your schedule.

Bottom line, technostress manifests itself in each and every one of us to various degrees. It is not a matter of "if" but rather "when" a technological glitch nails you and your ability to cope. Problem solving makes the difference in the degree of perceived hassle.

I have one more question that has not been answered regarding whether technostress is a passing problem or continuous future concern for the future generations. Today's children have grown up in the information age, so will there always be the problem of information overload with increasing availability of information sources and ways to access the sources, including upgrades, enhancements, and newer and better hardware and software? My belief is that technology is not the problem but rather the issue of our brain's capacity to manage time and expectations in an unpredictable technological environment. In order to be at the top of our game, technology should be viewed as a sport, which requires conditioning, cross training, proper nutrition, and recovery time for both the mind and body.

THE MULTITASKING BRAIN

Take a moment and think about all of the things you are doing right now—obviously you are reading this article, but chances are good that you are also doing several things at once.

Perhaps you're also listening to music, texting a friend, checking your email in another browser tab or playing a computer game.

If you are doing several different things at once, then you may be what researchers refer to as a "heavy multitasker." And you probably think that you are fairly good at this balancing act. According to a number of different studies, however, you are probably not as effective at multitasking as you think you are.

In the past, many people believed that multitasking was a good way to increase productivity. After all, if you're working on several different tasks at once, you're bound to accomplish more, right? Recent research, however, has demonstrated that that switching from one task to the next takes a serious toll on productivity. Multitaskers have more trouble tuning out distractions than people who focus on one task at a time. Also, doing so many different things at once can actually impair cognitive ability.

What the Research on Multitasking Suggests

First, let's start by defining what we mean when we use the term *multitasking*. It can mean performing two or more tasks simultaneously, or it can also involve switching back and forth from one thing to another. Multitasking can also involve performing a number of tasks in rapid succession.

In order to determine the impact of multitasking, psychologists asked study participants to switch tasks and then measured how much time was lost by switching. In one study conducted by Robert Rogers and Stephen Monsell, participants were slower when they had to switch tasks than when they repeated the same task.

Another study conducted in 2001 by Joshua Rubinstein, Jeffrey Evans and David Meyer found that participants lost significant amounts of time as they switched between multiple tasks and lost even more time as the tasks became increasingly complex.

Understanding What the Multitasking Research Means

In the brain, multitasking is managed by what are known as mental executive functions. These executive functions control and manage other cognitive processes and determine how, when and in what order certain tasks are performed. According to researchers Meyer, Evans and Rubinstein, there are two stages to the executive control process. The first stage is known as "goal shifting" (deciding to do one thing instead of another) and the second is known as "role activation" (changing from the rules for the previous task to rules for the new task).

Switching between these may only add a time cost of just a few tenths of a second, but this can start to add up when people begin switching back and forth repeatedly. This might not be that big of a deal in some cases, such as when you are folding laundry and watching television at the same time. However, if you are in a situation where safety or productivity are important, such as when you are driving a car in heavy traffic, even small amounts of time can prove critical.

Practical Applications for Multitasking Research

Meyer suggests that productivity can be reduced by as much as 40 percent by the mental blocks created when people switch tasks. Now that you understand the potential detrimental impact of multitasking, you can put this knowledge to work to increase your productivity and efficiency.

Of course, the situation plays an important role. The costs of switching tasks while texting a friend and watching a football game probably are not going to cause any major problems. However, that fraction of a second it takes to change tasks could mean life or death for someone driving down the interstate while trying to find a good radio station or talking on the phone.

The next time you find yourself multitasking when you are trying to be productive, take a quick assessment of the various things you are trying to accomplish. Eliminate distractions and try to focus on one task at a time.

7

Technological Addiction

Teens, Parents and the New Family Unit

In the words of Katie Pinholster an amazingly intuitive psychologist, who specializes in helping adolescents, parents, and families, "Addiction is addiction." Ultimately all addictive processes allow the brain to numb the things we prefer not to deal with. But are we addicted to our technological devices? Let's face it, in todays fast paced society technology gives us the chance to have killer lives, helping us control our schedules, handle clients, family, and friends from around the world. Yet due to this modern day marvel of technological devices we find ourselves fielding a communication conundrum that affects our work and personal life at all hours of the day and night. The latest crisis affecting life is knowing when to turn it off. Our brains are confronted by emails, text, voice mails, tweets, and other forms of social media, which redefine the psychological traits that make us human. Catherine Steiner-Adair Author of *The Big Disconnect* states, "Technology is redefining the fundamental cues, content, and cadence of our communication and the improvisational, uniquely human dimension of connection." Neuroscience confirms that our devices tap into the part of our brain that seeks order, pushing our need to be in control, organized and able to respond immediately. Our brain starts to react to these digital demands as necessary, prompting an impulsive response to everybody, anytime and anywhere. With the worlds acceptance of this compulsive behavior researchers have found that the time we spend on our devices gives us infinite access to life while eroding the traditional concept of how we connect and communicate with others.

The drama of the world is the same, it's just the format has changed. While the human brain, as we know it is starting to change due to its interaction with technology. Winifred Gallagher in her book *RAPT*, talks about life being the sum of what you focus on. Meaning the brains expanding capability and desire to connect to technological devices is without a doubt redefining the concept of family, relationships and choices. Our devices perpetuate the illusion of better life and a happier more fulfilling reality. We extinguish the present moment by diving into the abyss of the Internet and social media. These techno devices impart a distorted mental landscape with a sense of urgency to react the same way we instinctually need to eat, drink, and engage in sex. These devices have become surrogate body parts that give each and everyone of us 24/7 access to unlimited information, people, places and entertainment. Technological devices are an essential part of contemporary society playing a critical role in lives of young and old. Regardless how technology may change collectively it will continue to provide each person a space to connect with corporations, business associates, like minded communities, friends, family, and many times individuals that you would have never met. If you watch Mad Men, reruns of Ozzie and Harriet or My Three Sons, there was a time when families visited other families, kids congregated at their favorite spots, and business meetings (international and national) took place face to face. Although this still happens, the introduction of technology combined with social media has redefined today's external and internal world. This technological shift has enabled the integration of social and cultural factors that allow anyone to visit anywhere on the globe without physically transporting oneself anywhere, if they have the right device, app, Web address, or email. Technology has given each one of us the ability to participate in or help create our own world by reshaping our information landscape and the way we communicate. The application of technology readily creates new spaces for people to come together, connect and restructure relationships that share the same interest, activity or purpose. These amazing addictive devices have altered are sense of space, time and imagination, allowing individuals to reintroduce themselves into a broader audience attached to an expansive world.

How should we define techno addiction? As an everyday for instance, when scientists suggest our favorite food is addictive due to palatability, they are referring primarily to its capacity to stimulate the appetite and prompt us to eat more. The concept of palatability involves the brain's motivation to pursue a desired taste and is based on how the preferred food engages our full range of senses. And it is that stimulus that encourages a given response. Technology has its own palatability that leverages the techno addict's appetite making information more spreadable. Knowledge about a specific subject or situation is not new yet what is new is the means used to deliver this information. These technological devices give each person the capability to alter and amplify any situation, which offers the info-consuming techno addict technical features that introduce modes of communication that lead to well-established mental patterns of behavior. Like our favorite food, technology possesses intrinsic power over the brain's neurological pathways affecting all people who use it. So are we addicts to our devices, probably not, but the brain of the human species does have a strong need to develop meaningful relationships. Technology gives an individual the capacity to consciously create and recreate their digital presence for different purposes. For many individuals, technological devices fill that gap in one's life whether it is loneliness, information gathering, news related to recent events, or the need to get sound advice or counseling. But the next question is why does everyone seem to so intimately connect in an unhealthy way to his or her smartphone, tablet and laptop? Are we addicts or simply socially motivated and focused when we find ourselves perpetually texting? As one mom said to me, "What makes me crazy is when my daughter is upstairs and instead of coming downstairs to tell me she is ready to go somewhere, she texts me." When we refer to widespread technological addiction, are we actually making a factual statement regarding an unhealthy relationship with technological devices or are we just trying to stay connected to our world through the use of technology and social media?

These devices give us a means to join public spaces on the Internet, access to celebrities, special interest groups, and the latest scoop on anyone, anyplace, and at any time of the day or night. My clients tell me that they would rather meet people face to face, but their lives are out of control with crazy personal, family and business obligations. Bottom line is that everyone seems to be overly scheduled, even my dermatologist told me she triple books to assure maximal profitability, career satisfaction, and the expenses of a second home and kids in college.

I have been told that going online is like having a glass of Merlot or Pinot Noir, giving each person's brain the opportunity to escape their real life situation and many times find acceptance in online communities like Facebook, LinkedIn, Twitter, Pinterest and other socially networked communities. As a personal example, every evening when I walk in the door I find my husband Jeff surfing eBay, Amazon, car and motorcycle sites, Audi World, Huffington Post, The Daily Show, you name it he is on it. Our identities don't require a physical form anymore just a digital format. If we are in fact addicts of the digital age then we are all addicts. Liken us to drug addicts that share needles, we influence one another with new sites and help others by collectively engaging in creating the next most popular site to visit. This is a social process; with all this being said, like any unwanted pattern of behavior, some people absolutely develop unhealthy relationships within the world of technology. Any obsession can drastically affect your life. So where do we draw the line calling it a pathology. Pathological behavior is a mental or physical condition happening regularly, and seemingly impossible to control. It seems an over simplification to shift the problems of life tagging it "Techno Addiction." Are addictions simply bad? Addiction to alcohol was rampant in the so-called cradle of civilization 3,000 BCE. The Indians, Assyrians and Egyptians were addicted to opium poppy. 1200 CE, the Incas used the leaves of coca used for cocaine as payment for goods and services. In the 15th century ancient Greeks used a form of fermented honey called mead or beer to induce visions. Sir Walter Raleigh introduced the New World to a more fashionable, socially acceptable addictive drug, tobacco and by the 17th century numerous drugs were traded worldwide. Let's not forget the 1960's and peyote, fly agaric and cannabis. Then there is the lure of Las Vegas and the state lotteries encouraging us to gamble responsibility. Hey my grandmother was addicted to gardening, my sister to equestrian wear and horses, and my son gambles on line with fantasy football. And I have clients addicted to everything from Jimmy Choo shoes to tennis and others to BARRE classes, so exactly where do we draw the line. The truth is our brains enjoy these neurochemical ebbs and flow, hits and fixes whether we are surfing a technological devices or fixated on some other product, app or website.

Are we addicted or could it be we just don't know how to set boundaries. It is well established by the number of traffic fatalities that we compulsively check our smartphones and text while driving. We don't feel whole if we leave home without our tablet or cell, we sleep with them like a love interest, addicted to the ping, the possibility of an email, Facebook, or a simple tweet. Yet, we continue to handle these devices while telling others how addictive they are; the tech effect has transformed every part of our daily life from the moment we rise to the moment we hit the sheets.

But are we truly addicted? Addiction was initially reserved for the use of drug and alcohol abuse but over time this term has come to represent any unwanted behavior. Techno addiction was categorized under behavioral compulsion, which means an impulse-control disorder. I feel the notion of addiction has been modernized, homogenized and taken out of its initial context. I have found people can over do anything from running to coffee. An addiction is an addiction only if its use impedes ones ability to lead a healthy productive life. Danah Boyd's author of *It's Complicated,* hit the nail on the head when she stated, "The problem with popular discussions about addiction is that it doesn't matter whether people are chemically or psychologically dependent on a substance or behavior. Anyone who engages in a practice in ways that society sees as putting more socially acceptable aspects of their lives in jeopardy are seen as addicted." I guess it comes down to determining whether your brain's craving is socially acceptable or not. In today's world every man, women, young adult, teen, tween, and child has a busy schedule and compressed time needs. How many more opportunities can we manage to jam into our already hyper active lives?

Why should we consider separating our digital lives from our actual life? Our devices allow us an unending affair with social media. Every person on the planet with an internet connection now has the opportunity to socialize with friends, create or join a community of like-minded individuals, people watch, get a degree, attend a conference, meeting or webinar on line without leaving work or the comfort of home. In fact, access to the Internet has lifted most physical restriction for the handicapped, and those who are too young or too old. If we are talking about an addiction to the available dialogue and information on the internet we are condemning a curious yet healthy desire to be aware of what is going on in the world, in are cities, neighborhoods, schools, churches, government, and people in general.

The real question is, are we ready to embrace the inevitable changes that technology has wrapped around the human brain and its neuropathways? We know that some aspects of technology are addictive and that different types of brains are more vulnerable than others. Our brains, though vincible have kept pace with every new invention from the printing press, radio, television, movies, and now the Internet. Pathologizing technology, ignoring or micro managing the inevitable future will not make us more responsible for the use of technology or its other resources unless we are given the time to learn how to become evolved stewards. Let's recognize that the Internet has become a global tool that provides us a window into society allowing connectivity through the exploration of worldwide networks made up of diverse places attached to many different and varied types of elements, forms, content and individuals. Within this digital presence there seems to be a sense of heritability of characteristics that implies how these networks form. Given that social networks play a critical role in determining the future on a variety of topics ranging from global catastrophic events to the lives of the rich and famous, it is critically important that we grasp how these technological networks exhibit the patterns they do when they exercise influence over the world's populations. Researchers have well established that personal characteristics and behavior play critical roles in determining who interacts with whom. To some degree genetic traits may influence individuals in terms of their predisposition regarding like tendencies of social network groups. The significance of genetics influencing the formation of networks is of substantial interest and suggests a potential starting point for a deeper understanding of how we can manage behavior. It seems that in studies surrounding social network characteristics heritability can influence how likely someone is to initiate or accept the premise of new beliefs or patterns and behaviors. Yet this notion of heritability can't directly impact the degree of acceptance nor how likely a given individual will respond to the change message. As a global society it is time to recognize what each and every one of us is trying to achieve and work responsibly within this dynamic technological landscape with a sense of life-work balance and mindfulness regarding the worlds technological resources. Humankind has a unique opportunity and responsibility to shape this new technological and cultural landscape. What lies ahead is no more than a rumor yet what we do know is that technology and it's online social networking is the future of business, education, marketing, recruiting, product development and relationships. Technology and online social media is a new breed of animal that is waiting to be understood and used for the betterment of mankind. Catherine Steiner-Adair, EdD, author of *The Big Disconnect* reminds us as a species the use of technology is incapable of replacing our values, information, context, community and it surely cannot provide direct, nourishing, and uniquely human dimension of relationships essential for healthy neurological and psychological development.

Regardless of all this banter, if we do not ultimately control what we have created, technology will continue to transform the brain, life and its interpretation, with or without our consent. We are the architects of our own technological landscapes. Technology is a game changer and perception shifter that will give us the chance to explore the unforeseen future state of the planet and the edges of the human brain.

8

The Hunger Brain

Forging a New Relationship With Food

Are we simply subjected to a "Toxic Food Environment" or are we dealing with the obesity epidemic as an addictive brain disease? Every morning hundreds of Americans walk past a vending machine on their way to their office. Some barely notice the distraction. Others, however, stop and peer into the volume of eye candy to see what grabs their craving and taste interest. They pull out their money, insert the correct change, take the specific food, and munch on it on the way to their desk or meeting. The next day, they round the corner, see the vending machine, remember that incredible taste, and as if on autopilot pull out the correct change, take the food of choice and again eat it on the way to their office. Whether walking past the vending machine, driving through a fast food establishment that offers your favorite breakfast special or a coffee shop with the best latte, this is how the simple pleasure of a specific food creates addictive patterns in the brain. But are individuals really on their way to becoming addicts? Mike Dow, Pd.D., and Clinical Director of Therapeutic and Behavioral services of the Body Well Integrative Medical Center in Los Angeles has said openly that the addiction to food can be harder to overcome than drugs and that food addictions are just as real as drug and alcohol addictions.

It has been over two decades since the October 1993 edition of Vegetarian Times stated that, "Surveys have suggested that anywhere from 20 to 70 percent of Americans say the urge for a certain food sometimes strike them." In the past year regardless of race or socio-economic class, surveys estimate almost 100% of young women and nearly 70% of young men report having experienced cravings. America has become imprisoned by food cravings and obesity, the modern health epidemic of today's world. It is believed the reason most diets fail is that they don't address the changes in brain chemistry caused by food that can be more powerful than the effects of cocaine. Researchers and scientists at the National Institute of Drug Abuse (NIDA) have been trying to figure out whether we truly can be addicted to food by studying the brains reaction with high-tech scanners. And what they can say is that the brain of an obese person looks similar to the brain of a drug addict. In the world of endless foods, many diets work in practice yet are unhealthy in theory. Study after study alludes to the fact that the high prevalence of craving behaviors in today's global economy has created a negative nutritional impact and has been linked to snacking behavior, poor diet compliance, and the continuing rise in the obesity rate. Virtually everyone has or will at some point, experience a food craving which is expressed as a pressing desire to taste a very particular food. The image associated with the word craving depicts deprivation, starvation, extreme hunger and temptation. The desire to eat hyper-palatable foods come down to 50 percent genetics and the rest to environmental factors like cheap, calorie-dense, fast food, junk food and super sized portions for pennies more. Over time the strengthening of the brain's neural pathways for a particular food along with a sharp rise in dopamine and serotonin (neurochemicals that affect the brain's pleasure centers) makes forgoing one's favorite food unbearable and completely unthinkable. There is another form of reinforcement, an arousal of wanting more. So what came first the chicken or the egg?

The traditional diet deals with two factors—calorie consumption and restriction. This approach to food leads to short-lived successes because of its failure to address the pitfalls associated with the brain's conditioning for a specific food, taste, texture, and smell. Even researchers remain unclear whether a legitimate physiological basis for intense desires for certain foods truly exists, citing difficulty in isolating psychological, social, and cultural factors that play a strong role in food choices. What researchers do agree upon is that food cravings come from the same part of the brain as an addict's. When studying craving, researchers have used functional magnetic resonance imaging to reveal that food cravings activate brain areas related to emotion, memory and reward —which are the same areas activated during drug addiction studies. The pattern of MRI results suggests that the memory area of the brain responsible for associating a food with a reward are more important to food craving than are the actual reward centers or hunger itself. This is consistent with the idea that cravings of all kinds, whether for food, drugs, cars or designer shoes, all share the same common mechanisms. Marcia Levin Pelchat, at the Monell Chemical Senses Center feels if we ever hope to get a handle on the craving cycle, we need to learn much more about food cravings in pathological conditions such as obesity, alcoholism, cocaine addiction and other drug conditions. Marcia Pelchat stated, "Since so many of these excesses of desire share common brain mechanisms, then it may be seen as plausible that motivational trade-offs could be developed to treat cravings with a healthier substitute." Pelchat makes the point you can label craving behavior as excessive hunger, a desire for a specific food, emotional eating, or an addiction; in the end, it leads to your demise, forcing you to eat more.

A far more persuasive finding by Adam Drewnowski, at the University of Washington in Seattle, parallels the same physiological mechanisms involved in food cravings as for an addict's desire for opiates. Drewnowski, who has spent thirty years studying human taste, food preferences, and dietary choices, found that the opioid circuitry, which is the body's primary pleasure system, created a similar effect to drugs like morphine and heroin. Opioid produced by the consumption of high-sugar, high-fat foods can relieve and disrupt pain or stress in the body. Drewnowski's studies show that with infusions of various opiate-blockers, preferences for foods high in fat and sugar decrease. He speculates that opiate blockers interfere with the ability to experience pleasure, including the pleasure derived from the tastes and textures of food.

The face of food addiction varies from person to person. For some, craving may be that sugary pick-me-up or a bag of salt/pepper potato chips, a couple pieces of your favorite chocolate, or the extra glass of wine at night to unwind from the day. The good news is that these types of unhealthy urges can be fended off. Science points to the validated fact that cravings seem to be all about blood sugar levels. Food cravings mean that the body has its signals mixed-up; it has nothing to do with willpower, yet developing "will power" is a skill base, not a myth or genetic trait. Do some individuals overeat because they were born with a non-responsive dopamine system or does the obese individual have a low dopamine response because they overeat, or could obesity itself weaken the dopamine system triggering over stimulation? All these scenarios promote weight gain leading researchers to believe we probably have low blood sugar or low serotonin levels, signaling the brain that it needs a burst of energy. Researchers like Susan Schiffman, Ph.D., professor of medical psychology at Duke University Medical Center, believes the "carbohydrate" craving cycle could simply be from hunger driven by blood sugar levels being too low, making such craving physiological in nature. A reoccurring viewpoint amongst researchers have found, if the individual's sugar levels stay constant throughout the course of the day, then eating patterns and consumption levels will be more controllable. Conversely, when times get chaotic, schedules overwhelming, and the individual doesn't get a food infusion for hours, the body's physiological and psychological stress levels begin to climb. One's blood sugar takes a nosedive for the worse and that craving for that favorite comfort food starts screaming your name. Researchers have targeted those favorite foods as the "high-carbohydrate demonic" food group. These high-carbohydrate foods also referred to as re- fined carbs or high-glycemic foods, increase levels of your brain's neurotransmitter called serotonin.

Kessler's explains carbohydrate cravings as a feedback mechanism between carbohydrates (sugar) and serotonin (plea- sure hormone). Neuroscientists talk about the mechanics of crav- ing behavior like this: when we eat a food high in refined sugar, fat, or salt, we stimulate neurons (cells in the brain). Then the neurons start to connect in circuits and communicate about the food eaten, which is referred to as "encoding" or "mental im- print." The neuron records a preference for that particular food creating an automatic response. David A. Kessler, MD, former FDA commissioner and author of *"The End of Overeating"*, refers to the brain's imprinting as an "action schemata", representing the specific sequence and actions taken in response to a desired palatable food. Kessler says that once a food script becomes im- printed in the brain, the behavior dictated becomes so routine that we respond automatically before we are even conscious of a stimulus. In fact, according to Howard Fields, a professor of neu- rology and physiology at the University of California, San Fran- cisco, a small proportion of neurons are "uniquely encoded to respond to a single sensory characteristic of food and stimulated by sight, smell, temperature and taste, texture, sweet, salty, sour, or bitter. Neurons react to foods by way of electrical signals that in turn release brain chemicals that then travel to other intercon- nected neurons that create the craving behavior."

And why is it that cravings seem to be experienced when we are exhausted or simply feeling blue? This feel good hormone is a brain neurotransmitter that some researchers suggest regu- lates carbohydrate intake, calming the brain, giving you that laid back, relaxed, everything will be "OK" feeling. Unfortunately these particular foods release a short burst of serotonin allowing us to feel good for a brief moment, before we get thrown into a low-serotonin state. These roller coaster highs lead to punishing downward spirals represented by a ravenous hunger that only another high-fat, high-sugar meal will satisfy. Richard Foltin, of Columbia University's department of Psychiatry, refers to this cycle thusly "real-factor comes down to sensory stimulation plus calorie stimulation. The relationship between human motivation and behavior in the presence of hyper-palatable food is still unraveling, but what we do know for certain is that foods high in sugar, fat, and salt are altering the biological circuitry of our brains.

Other thought leaders in the field of neuroscience and nutrition suggest that raising the level of serotonin, by consuming a high- carbohydrate meal satisfies a need and reduces the urge to eat more carbohydrates. Conversely, a high protein meal creates a serotonin deficit, which awakens the carbohydrate craving, leading to the consumption of foods high in carbohydrates. Yet most research takes the viewpoint that the more a dieter tries to restrict or lower the intake of carbohydrates (your most readily available source of energy), the more it seems that the craving takes hold and the diet effort fades away. Other factors associated with food cravings are connected to one's stress and hormone levels, sleep cycle, and mood.

Like the research of David A. Kessler, the majority of researchers maintain the mindset that people's food choices are probably influenced by the brain's reactions prior to eating experiences. Scientists noted that when a food elicits top mental performance, the brain keeps an internal food journal of preferred foods for making future choices. Another supporter of the "prior eating experience scenario" is Linda Bartoshuk, PH.D in Psychology at Yale University, who has stated "The brain has the ability to make associations with food eaten for the first time, deciding whether or not the food eaten provided a benefit, like a boost of energy or a warm, fuzzy feeling". Familiarity begets acceptability, and acceptability begets cravings. It has become fact that humans crave things that they've had positive experiences with.

The craving script goes something like this—the first time

you have the experience or learn something new, chances are a new pathway is created and imprinted in your memory similar to saving it under "Favorites" on your computer. The next time that same experience or learning is reinforced because neurons that learn together become attached, the more often one experiences the same thought or behavior, and the stronger the neural pathway will become. All beliefs, behaviors, and assumptions are contained in your brain's neural pathways. Each time you have an experience; it is imprinted along these pathways sending electro-chemical messages to the brain. This is how we create habits good and bad.

A Lesson in Mental Performance

Let's say for example that Amy has a real desire for potato chips, she just loves the crunch and the taste of salt, which turns into her eating an entire bag. She has made every effort to stop this behavior yet, every time Amy opens a bag of chips, the smell and taste send her into a binging behavior, making it exponentially more difficult to stop the habituation.

If Amy really wants to change this behavior, the habit itself must be changed to alter the neural pathways. In order to implement and sustain real behavioral change, this gradual shift over time forces the existing neural pathways to weaken and atrophy. This is similar to not exercising, and your muscles become deconditioned. Basically, Amy is trying to override the old habit by rewiring the brain's pathways with a new behavior, experience or learning. The next step involves Amy practicing these new behaviors over and over till new pathways take hold.

Even Oprah's Mehmet C. Oz, M.D. author of *You on a Diet,* has a "factoid" in his book reinforcing the notion that emotional eating starts in the brain, which comes from your food memory. Oz points to the fact that chemicals in the brain influence our emotions and provide the foundation for why, what, and when we eat. Oz along with most scientists and PhD's believe what goes on in the brain plays a vital role in what happens to the waistline.

He and others believe the key to resisting those cravings lies in your ability to understand how emotions prioritize your eating patterns. Oz explains that when the level of serotonin in your brain falls, your body senses starvation that initiates the craving of carbs. A majority of researchers have a consistent theme, keep your brain happy by maintaining a steady state of your feel-good hormones serotonin.

Dr. Kelly Brownell, a psychologist at Yale University, has proposed the concept referred to as "Toxic Food Environment". In Brownell's work with the severely obese he found that the American diet is shaped by an extraordinary array of high-calorie, low-nutrient food, much of which has been carefully engineered to stimulate and then satisfy cravings. As a result, he feels the palate of an average person has been conditioned to a diet of high-fat, high-sugar, and high starch, which from a psychological standpoint is also highly addictive. Brownell believes we need to reprogram our chemistry from an unhealthy toxic food environment to foods designed by nature, in which the factors of appetite, metabolism, and food choices synergistically work together to create and maintain a healthy body weight.

Let's take a look at today's reality – many individuals are under a great deal of stress or suffer from insomnia, sleep deprivation, work nights, and feel exhausted most of the time. This leads to adrenal fatigue or outright exhaustion that signals the body that it needs a pick-me-up. You may resort to a sugary snack or a coffee, a high carb high fat meal, or a couple of alcoholic drinks at night, all of which exacerbate the problem. The fact that many Americans of all ages don't get enough sleep or recovery time escalates the reports of cravings, impaired immune systems, and increased risk of diseases from frequent colds, to diabetes or obesity. Another soldier in the war against obesity is David Levitsky, a professor of nutrition and psychology at Cornell University in Ithaca who seems to believe dieting increases the potential to crave when we restrict ourselves from certain food selections saying, "No, I can't eat this and I can't eat that". Levitsky, who has studied cravings combined with weight control for more than 25 years, says that the most craved foods are usually the highest in calories composed primarily of refined sugar and fat because that is exactly what dieters give up. Though there is an ongoing controversy over what diets seem to work best, researchers along with registered dietitians and nutritionists know that meals with a mix of lean protein, complex carbohydrate and low-fat provide just the right balance to support brain function. Researchers and scientists alike believe that high-carbohydrate diets composed of low-glycemic/complex carbohydrate food, may be the most successful because they work best with our brain chemistry. Since carbohydrates represent a major source of fuel for daily activities like thinking skills and muscular movements, severely limiting the amount of carbs consumed takes a toll on your overall performance.

Many studies claim age as another factor that affects cravings. The research of Marcia Levin Pelchat her article on Food Craving in Young and Elderly Adults, it seems individuals younger than 65 consistently say they crave specific foods more often than those older than 65. Scientists think that this is because the senses of smell and taste, which are strong appetite stimulants diminishes as we age. So how does a simple craving for French fries, ice cream, or brownies put us at such risk? The perpetuated cycle connected to craving goes something like this—a simple-refined variety of carbohydrate foods puts you in an "insulin-hunger" cycle causing your blood sugar levels to elevate then drop dramatically, which creates hunger pangs and intense cravings. When individuals are stressed (chemical, physical, emotional, neurological, environmental, or technological) their insulin and cortisol levels increase. In other words chronic elevated insulin levels can increase stress levels. And stress levels increase cortisol. And the more cortisol in your body, the higher your insulin level which in turn causes the body to store fat, resulting in those love handles or muffin tops you hate. This perpetuating cycle only gets worse as you blame yourself for eating senselessly which intensifies your mood increasing the need for more foods that will give you that feel good burst of energy.

The Common Thread

The common link in all of these theories is the hormone insulin which is responsible for maintaining your blood sugar within a narrow range, storing fat in your cells, sugar in your liver, and influences the expression of amino acids when building muscle. Under stress, cortisol commands your body to essentially ignore insulin's direction and instead to make sugar, fat, and amino acids available for conversion into glucose (sugar) that is your body's first line of energy. This causes cortisol to order your cells to stop taking in sugar, which increases the insulin in your bloodstream. This is defined as "insulin resistance". When cravings press your body into insulin resistance, you end up with too much insulin in the bloodstream, which forces the body to secrete more cortisol to balance the effects of too much insulin which creates weight gain derived from innocently eating a high carbohydrate meal. Scientists have found that a diet higher in protein and moderate in carbohydrates appear to modify the body's insulin signal by promoting control of insulin production and levels of blood glucose. The extreme rise and fall of one's blood sugar throughout the day, day after day, results in over stimulation of insulin in the bloodstream leading to today's health crisis called metabolic syndrome. Metabolic syndrome also referred to as insulin resistance syndrome or syndrome X, targets four risk factors in the development of cardiovascular disease – diabetes, obesity, hypertension, and high blood cholesterol. The research of Robert A. Hegele MD, affiliated with Blackburn Cardiovascular Genetic Laboratory and Robarts Research Institute and Department of Medicine points to the fact that individuals with metabolic syndrome may possess an underlying genetic predisposition that is expressed when poor diet and lack of exercise habits result in obesity.

After all the theorizing on why we crave or how we gain or lose weight, the question seems to focus on whether cravings have a scientific basis, or are they nothing more than personal quirks? There seems to be a growing body of evidence that accepting food cravings and keeping them in check may be the most important component of weight management. Cravings are not thought to cause people to become overweight. And when talking about craving, we are usually referring to the over consumption of a specific food. Overweight on the other hand, tends to come from small, sustained increases in food intake on a daily basis. On the end of the spectrum cravings aren't even believed to wreck weight loss diets, at least not diets that people are able to adhere to over the long haul. Researchers suggest that while people may be tempted by cravings when they first embark on a weight-loss plan, the cravings tend to wane over time. Even the initial craving can be minimized to a lesser degree by making sure the diet is not too monotonous. Studies seem to conclude that the fewer foods a person is allowed to consume, the more frequent and intense the cravings will tend to be. The train of thought in the field of dieting is if you are not trying to lose weight, or on a medically restricted diet, let the craving win. Otherwise you will probably do more psychological damage by defying the body's food preference.

The Science of Craveability and Your Weight

Accepting food cravings and keeping them in check may be an important component of weight management, according to findings from the first six-month phase of a calorie-restriction study conducted at the Jean Mayer USDA Human Nutrition Research Center on Aging (USDA HNRCA) at Tufts University. Supplemental results from the Comprehensive Assessment of the Long-term Effects of Restricting Intake of Energy (CALERIE) trial provide new insights into food cravings, specific types of foods craved, and their role in weight control. According to findings based on calorie-restriction conducted by Jean Mayer, dieters who occasionally gave in to cravings had the most weight-loss success. Susan Roberts, PhD., director of the USDA HNRCA's

Energy Metabolism Laboratory and her team observed that successful weight loss was tied not only to how often people gave in to their cravings, but also to the types of foods they craved. "Subjects with a higher percentage of weight loss actually craved foods with higher caloric density, compared with those who lost a lower percentage of body weight," says Roberts, who is also a professor at the Friedman School of Nutrition Science and Policy at Tufts University. "Energy-dense foods, such as chocolate and some salty snacks, are those that pack the most calories per unit of volume," explains Cheryl Gilroy, PhD, MPH, research dietitian and first author of the study, "as compared to less energy-dense foods like fruits and vegetables, which have fewer calories per unit of volume." Roberts findings suggest that food cravings are for calories, not necessarily carbohydrates calories, as is widely spread by word of mouth, magazines, supplement pushers, and diet books. What is commonly labeled as a carbohydrate addiction should probably be relabeled as calorie addiction. Some of the most commonly craved foods among studied participants were foods that were high in sugar, fat, and salt, such as chocolate, and salty snacks, chips and French fries. The biggest eye opener Roberts disclosed is that the most identifiable thing about the foods people crave are that they are highly dense in calories. As in the research of David A. Kessler, MD, author of *The End of Overeating*, who reported that the goals of the food industry are to get you hooked on what he identified as dense caloric foods composed of sugar, fat and salt. Kessler elaborates about the "craveability" factor explaining how the food industry intentionally layers the product with sauces, cheese and breading, which are cheaper to produce than the central ingredient such as meat or fish. What do we crave? Sweets first, then salty stuff of with both foods layered with fats.

COMMONLY CRAVED FOODS
- Alcohol
- Chicken wings
- Cheeseburger
- Chocolate
- Hamburger
- Ice cream
- Peanut butter
- Pickles
- Pie
- Pizza
- Potato chips
- Pretzels
- Soft drinks

Managing the Hunger Brain

The bottom line to reducing cravings begins with forging a new relationship with food. How we make food choices is a complex issue. Beyond the basic need to satisfy the brain's hunger, some of the most important physiological factors may be those of the food itself; characteristics of taste, texture, color, aroma and temperature. Our association with food and what particular foods signify in terms of the emotions they evoke clearly has a powerful influence. If you're going to break the crave cycle and escape your self-imposed prison of frustration and guilt associated with food, you will have to desensitize yourself to the foods you crave. In the final analysis, whether future research shows food cravings are physiologically based or psychologically based or both, targeting the desired food as the problem is a mistake. You will have to learn to kick those stubborn little urges to the curb and adopt a new, healthier attitude toward food instead of being derailed by your demonic attention combined with flimsy, limitless excuses.

Specific foods should not be labeled inherently good or bad, but rather foods that should be eaten in smaller amounts. You would be better off learning how to manage your cravings without indulging in high-carbohydrate, high-fat, salty foods.

Managing the Hunger Brain isn't the same thing as willpower. In every Hunger Brain there lies the heart of a hyper conditioned impulsive eater. Simply intellectualizing the right behavior isn't sufficient enough to protection one from food cues. The compulsive eater needs to develop a plan that will help prepare them for encounters with their favorite food. The implementation strategy is an awareness exercise to help redirect craving behaviors. The idea of planning gives the Hunger Brain a competitive advantage by enabling one to think through alternatives to their habitual eating patterns. When an implementation strategy is developed and employed, that will allow the Hunger Brain to better inhibit and redirect compulsive eating. A plan helps the Hunger Brain create new way of responding to food and clarifies the consequences associated with habitual behavior. Silvia Bunge, researcher at the University of Berkeley, believes the more specific the plan the easier it is for the Hunger Brain to practice the alternative actions to food cues and encounters. Practice make perfect when it comes to new behavior, new responses will eventually replace the unwanted behavior.

. Create a conscious cognitive script – a new strategy for your favorite foods. Researcher Silvia Bunge, PhD, head, Cognitive Control and Development Laboratory, UCB, suggest it is easiest to follow "categorical rules," like "I will not eat potato chips," " There will be no dessert or bread eaten at dinner," "I will eat one small serving of birthday cake at the party tonight."

. Be aware of your triggers – The smell, sound, texture or taste all become hunger cues. Researcher Pamela Peeke at the University of Maryland see the biggest rise in dopamine release when people are presented with different cues. Awareness is the first step towards change. Keep a record of all your favorite foods, write them down and describe why you like them and how they make you feel. Starting to evaluate a favorite food in a new way, helps protect you from it compelling emotional draw it has on your brain.

. Learn to manage stress – Stress acts as a distractor giving you permission to fall into the pattern of eating more of the foods you like. This is where comfort food got its name. Typically these favorite foods are jam packed with sugar, fat, and salt. Sadness and Anger have the greatest potential to drive a loss of control. Over time, neural pathways link the change in mood with the experience of eating your favorite food, creating a stronger urge.

. Redirect your attention – habit driven responses die-hard. Redirecting your focus offers you the capability to refuse the invitation to evoke the automatic food cue. If your favorite food becomes unavailable, it affects what you think and how you act, allowing you too more easily shift your attention. For instance when you recognize a consistent pattern of behavior like stopping a Starbucks daily for a Mocha Frappuccino you can change your traffic pattern by detouring your focus.

. Counter condition your brain—Change how you think about your favorite food, Philip David Zelazo of the University of Toronto, suggests altering our emotional appraisal of our favorite comfort food. Zelazo believes if we learn to view the pursuit of the undesirable food in a negative light and attach emotional significance to the unwanted behavior, it is possible to reverse the habit.

. Develop a meal plan – What foods you can eat, serving size, and time of day. Focus on your short-and long term health goals.

. Gauge your Hunger Brain – Start by waiting 30 minutes to assess how you feel on your hunger scale then once you conquer 30 minutes challenge your brain with 90 minutes. Remember the brain is a muscle needing constant cross training and conditioning. Eat only half of your usual meal. Wait 30 then 90 minutes and assess how you feel. You can practice eating by varying the serving size of your meal till you find what works for your hunger level.

. Eat Foods you enjoy – I know that sounds counter intuitive but it works. The enjoyment factor must be developed around the personal likes and dislikes. Eating is complicated, it is emotional, physical and contain genetic preferences in our brain due to a lifetime of experiences. Whether your preference is mostly protein, complex carbohydrates, or a green tea smoothie, success and control stems from your enjoyment of the preferred and permitted food.

. Exercise – Walk, run, treadmill, elliptical, stepper, and aerobic classes all can help to create new brain cells which in turn helps with working memory and the brain's cognitive reservoir. Aerobic activity generally increased the amount of dopamine receptors.

. Desirable behavior must be intrinsic in nature and have an emotional value that carries an incentive. And unless the Hunger Brain makes the cognitive shift in how it thinks, by reinforcing the benefits associated with a life "without a stimuli" verses life "with the stimuli" curbing overeating and developing self-control for the long haul is not possible. Research on craving and addiction is gaining traction.

. Forget forcing yourself to eat raw veggie or foods you just hate and instead have a reasonable serving size of your favorite comfort food. In moderation your favorite high calorie food can actually help you stay within a well-balanced diet while maintaining a healthy weight. Cravings do not have to defeat your weight-loss efforts. Those who do the best at weight loss don't lose their cravings; they just get better at managing them. You can't help being hardwired to yearn for sugar, fat or salt yet you can minimize the damage by replacing those calorie-dense foods with light versions of the same flavors you crave most.

When your eating habits are dominated by "shouldn't", it is time for a change. It is not a matter of "if" but "when" your willpower runs out of steam, remember you are simply having an impulse moment. This means you can react to a craving without a continuous stream of "mindless eating". Although the act of eating seems random, these cravings are activated by cues in our environment, aromas, commercials, thoughts, feelings, events and situations. In Dr. Phil McGraw's book *The Ultimate Weight Solution,* he talks about the "Impulse Moments" as critical for you to manage, because they can and will derail even the best of weight loss plans and efforts. And if you fail to get a grip on these daily impulses, which everyone gets, then you are going to go spiraling back into your habitually self-destructive eating behaviors every time.

Not everyone in the field of nutrition agrees that we can be addicted to this toxic food environment, and they object to the continuous excuses that fuel a billion dollar business. Let's stop shifting the blame of why we are unable to control the rate of obesity in this country and focus on being substance independent. And if indeed this epidemic resembles that of alcohol and drug addiction let's determine treatments for those addicted versus those who simply experience an occasional craving.

9

Euphoric Alcohol's Effect on Your Brain

To Drink or Not to Drink

An innocent sip of your favorite glass of wine or cocktail seems harmless enough…right? But research now shows that those innocent sips can wallop your mental and physical well-being. Alcohol is not just an energy source; it is a psychoactive drug and a toxin to the body. Ethanol (alcohol) is defined as the alcohol found in alcoholic beverages, produced by the action of microorganisms in the absence of oxygen on the carbohydrates of grape or other carbohydrate-containing fluids. When examining ethanol, it is less toxic than other varieties of alcohol when sufficiently diluted and taken in small enough doses.

Regardless, the benefits of alcohol's medicinal properties are mentioned 191 times in the Old and New Testaments. Yet when you ask for a drink, you've asked for a narcotic. Now your saying to yourself, that is crazy talk; how can that be? The category narcotic represents a drug that dulls the senses and induces sleep—a drug that in moderate doses dulls one's awareness and relieves pain but in excessive doses causes stupor, coma, or convulsions. Those being the facts, people have used alcohol for centuries as an anesthetic because it can deaden pain. Unfortunately it makes a poor anesthetic because you cannot predict how much each person will need and how much an individual can actually tolerate. Mankind has known the effects of wine, beer, and other fermented beverages for over 5000 years.

In today's contemporary society alcohol provides most individuals with the ability to "unwind" from the stressors of career and family. And it is well documented and researched that "if" taken in "moderation," alcohol relaxes the brain, reduces inhibitions, and encourages desirable social interaction. The scientific community views alcohol as an organic compound containing hydroxyl (OH) groups. A good example is glycerol, a sweet syrupy alcohol, obtained from fatty acids that serves as the backbone for triglycerides (one of the three main classes of dietary fat) and is utilized by the body as a lipid solvent. This syrupy solution has the ability to dissolve the lipids (fat, oil, phospholipids, and sterols) right out of your cell membranes which allows alcohol to penetrate the body's cells, rapidly killing microbial cells which also allows this compound to be considered a useful disinfectant. This is just one of the reasons why alcohols are considered toxic.

The real reason your reading this article is to determine "how much" can one have to drink. Am I right? So let's move on. It has been researched, verified, validated and written about over the years, and a drink is defined as 12 ounces of beer, 4 to 5 ounces of wine, 10 ounces of wine cooler, or 1 ounce of an 80 proof distilled spirit (whiskey, scotch, rum, or vodka).

For every article you read about the benefits of alcohol consumption, you will find one warning you about the risks associated with alcohol. A drink is any alcoholic beverage that delivers ½ ounce of pure ethanol and the actual amount a person can drink responsibly depends on genetics, health condition, gender, weight, age, and family history. Though moderate alcohol use seems to have some benefits, exceeding the two drinks a day for men and one drink a day for women changes the benefit to health risk ratio. Then if you are over 65 the rules change yet again. With the increase of age, adults break down of alcohol is at a slower rate, leading to intoxication quicker and for a longer period of time.

Myth   Alcohol is legal; therefore it is not a drug.
Truth   Alcohol is legal, but it alters body functions and is medi-
        cally defined as a narcotic or depressant drug.

Some individuals argue it can't be a narcotic because it's not regulated; well it is. There is driving under the influence (DUI) and driving while intoxicated (DWI), in either case drunk driving impairs the driver's ability which defines driving a motor vehicle with blood levels of alcohol in excess of a legal limit. That seems pretty regulated to me. In most jurisdictions a measurement such as a blood alcohol content in excess of a defined level, such as 0.05% or 0.08% defines the offense, with no need to prove impairment or being under the influence of alcohol. It takes about an hour and a half to metabolize one drink, depending on a person's body size, previous drinking experience, how recently the person has eaten, gender, age and the person's current health status.

A good idea is to eat something before drinking. Unlike alcohol, food requires time for digestion, which gives your alcoholic beverage less opportunity to penetrate the wall of your stomach, allowing a diffused and delayed effect on the brain. Drinking on an empty stomach not only causes an individual to feel the effects of alcohol immediately, but also brings about a higher blood alcohol level for a longer period of time and allows maximum anesthesia to the brain. You really do not want a D.U.I do you?

Working at a country club and corporate wellness center gives a Wellcoach like myself a broad and varied perspective on the use and abuse of alcohol consumption. I have witnessed how alcohol can shift your behavior up close and personal with my athletes and weekend warriors only to recognize how commonplace having a few drinks has become. Then there is this powerful ongoing misconception in the news and on television that exercise can offset three straight nights of copious drinking. When adding the fitness factor to alcohol consumption, many times people allude to the notion of "sweating out" all the toxins associated with alcohol combined with poor eating habits and recreational drugs.

Let's get it right from the start. Alcohol consumption can be down right lethal and toxic to the body, not only because it depends on one sole organ, the liver, but because metabolism is slower than its consumption. This means most of the calories consumed during a single sitting move straight into fat generation and storage because alcohol cannot be made into an energy source or stored as a carbohydrate. However, because of how it operates in the body during its breakdown it ends up impacting fat storage. Alcohol is broken down into acetaldehyde and eventually acetate, which is similar to vinegar. The metabolite acetaldehyde interferes with protein formation, such as those involved in blood clotting. Then there are the increased levels of alcohol consumption, which lead to an accumulation of ammonia, which is toxic to the brain. Numerous nutritional studies find that heavy drinking is most responsible for the increased development of risk factors associated with metabolic syndrome, which parallels the current obesity epidemic. The undesired outcome of having too many drinks is exhibited by increases in waist circumference (or girth), triglycerols (fatty acids), blood pressure, and blood glucose levels. It can go without saying not only is alcohol toxic to the body; it is without a doubt seriously detrimental to your waistline.

ALCOHOL and FITNESS

Working in a fitness center for three decades has allowed me to witness first hand how drinking affects a work out. Research shows the role alcohol plays in the rate of injury and performance. In fact, chronic alcohol use affects muscle fiber size, decreasing capillary infusion into the muscle, thus affecting circulation. Here is a myth you have heard for years; a shot of alcohol warms you up. The truth is alcohol diverts blood flow to the skin making you feel warmer, but it actually cools the body. Alcohol simply blunts the good intentions of exercise, health and wellness. Individuals engaging in intense exercise and intense drinking create much more physiological damage not to mention the increased risk of metabolic syndrome, estrogen dominance, tissue inflammation and detrimental protein degradation.

Yet, sports and alcohol seem to have a longstanding relationship amongst professional athletes, team sports, weekend warriors, and recreational exercisers. It is not like there are no studies out there to review. A study on "feminization" associated with chronic alcohol abuse published in the Journal of Steroid Biochemistry (1988), evaluated wine drinkers versus beer drinkers. The outcome indicated fast beer drinkers, a practice prevalent among many recreational weekend exercisers, experienced significant elevation of blood estradiol otherwise known as estrogen, and depressed testosterone levels. There exists evidence that alcohol and metabolites actually affect the body's hormonal make-up which means if a male increases his drinking level or becomes a chronic drinker, he will begin to show signs of feminization, resulting basically from an increased estrogen production, as opposed to testosterone which kind of defeats the desired outcome of building muscle mass during intense weight training. These facts reveal that the effects of alcohol abuse outweigh the beneficial hormonal effects of resistance training. Other studies published in Medicine and Science in Sports and Exercise (2005), found that heavy alcohol use significantly reduced testosterone receptors that impact the fast twitch muscle fibers and a moderate effect on the slow twitch fibers. This doesn't represent a real problem for females but definitely is not a good thing for men who want to intensify their weight-training workout.

Basically, whether male or female, if you're deciding to engage in intense exercise combined with intense drinking, there is no upside to achieving a fit physique. Chronic drinking can only serve to deliver an array of physiological damage.

INSIDE THE BODY

Let's look inside the human body. The liver is the sole organ in the human body that can dispose of significant quantities of alcohol. The notion of your brain sobering up through drinking caffeine products or sweating it out through exercise cannot metabolize alcohol. The liver uses two processes to rid your body of alcohol, first is an enzyme referred to as ADH or alcohol dehydrogenase, tasked with removal of hydrogen from alcohol and break it down which accounts for about 80 percent. Then there is a chain of enzymes called MEOS known as microsomal ethanol oxidizing system which is charged with oxidizing not only 10 percent of all the alcohol you drink but several other classes of drugs. The remaining 10 percent is excreted through breath and urine.

Moving on to a dietary perspective, alcohol derived from alcoholic beverages slows down the body's use of fat for fuel by as much as 33 1/3 percent, causing more fat to be stored. The storage of fat is primarily visceral fat tissue stored within the abdominal cavity, which translates to around the middle or thighs and legs. Therefore alcohol consumption on top of a person's normal caloric consumption of food is fattening both through the calories (7 calories per gram) and through its effect on fat metabolism. The reason is that ethanol is a much less complicated molecule, super easy to digest and absorb fast so it's given the red carpet treatment the moment you take that first melodious sip. In fact, it gets absorbed and metabolized before most medications and nutrients. Then to worsen the whole drinking experience, 20 percent of the substance is absorbed right through the walls of an empty stomach, which gives alcohol access to the brain in a New York minute. It would be wise to "think" before you reach for a glass of euphoric delight and eat a high-fat snack. High fat foods generally help to keep the alcohol in your stomach longer, this is why food establishments put peanuts and those cute little fish in front of you when they serve you that martini. Of course there is a secondary reason for the "no charge snacks," they are full of sodium and make you thirsty.

Moving on, once alcohol reaches the stomach, it begins to break down with the alcohol dehydrogenase enzyme. Women produce less of this enzyme, which may help to partially explain why we become more intoxicated on less alcohol than men. As your drink travels through the stomach, it is rapidly absorbed in the upper portion of the small intestine. The alcohol-laden blood from the small intestines then travels to the liver via the veins and capillaries of the digestive tract, which affects nearly every liver cell. The liver cells are the only cells in our body that can produce enough of the enzyme alcohol dehydrogenase to oxidize alcohol at an appreciable rate.

Alcohol affects every organ of the body; its most dramatic impact is upon the liver due to its ability to filter the blood, remove and process nutrients, manufacture materials for export to other parts of the body, and destroy toxins or store them to keep them out of the circulation. The liver cells normally prefer a diet of fatty acids as fuel, and package excess fatty acids as triglycerides (fat), which they then route to other tissues within the body. However, when alcohol is present, the liver cells are directed to first metabolize the alcohol, letting the fatty acids accumulate, sometimes in huge amounts. Listen closely; cause I don't want to mince my words, alcohol metabolism permanently changes liver cell structure, which impairs the livers ability to metabolize fats. This explains why heavy drinkers tend to develop what is known as a "fatty liver."

Unfortunately, the liver is able to metabolize about 1 ounce of ethanol per hour. Another way to think of it is it takes the body approximately an hour and a half to metabolize one drink. If more alcohol arrives in the liver than the enzymes can handle, the excess alcohol travels to all parts of the body, circulating until the liver enzymes are finally able to process it. Whether it is beer, wine or liquors, all confer the very same health effects. And what may you be asking yourself? Well, according to Eric Rimm, ScD, associate professor of nutrition at the School of Public Health at Harvard University, the French Paradox surrounding the heart friendly benefit of red wine as a health food due to its antioxidants is no longer the thought. More recent research has shown that antioxidants are not the answer. The ethanol in the alcohol raises levels of protective high-density lipoproteins (HDL, or good cholesterol), which is what helps protect against plaque buildup in the arteries and reduce clotting factors that contribute to heart attacks and stroke. Any kind of beverage that contains alcohol when consumed in moderation (one to two drinks a day) helps reduce the risk of heart disease.

A liver clogged with fatty acids cannot function properly. Liver cells become less efficient at performing a number of tasks, which impairs a person's nutritional health in a way that cannot be corrected with diet alone. To overcome problems associated with alcohol consumption, the individual needs to stop drinking for a while; otherwise the liver's inability to synthesize fatty acids accelerates the more you drink.

Alcohol is age resistant. Meaning age really doesn't matter to our old friend alcohol. Alcohol is smart as a whip and knows implicitly that our teens and young adults do not benefit by drinking; rather they increase the probability of dying from other causes such as car crashes, homicides, and other forms of violence. Alcohol's efficacy is just not equal for men, women, young, old and the health impaired and as for the wine consumption don't even get me started. The science on wine and health is mixed and comes down to who is paying for the comment.

ALCOHOL and the BRAIN

Regardless of the potential dangers associated with alcohol being given the status of a toxic narcotic, droves of the business sector, young singles, teens and moms with kids, the sick, aging and elderly, depressed and lonely individuals take a drink to relax or relieve anxiety. People honestly believe that alcohol is a stimulant because it seems to lower inhibitions, when in actuality it sedates or suppresses inhibitory nerves, which are more numerous than excitatory nerves. This makes alcohol a depressant, which affects all the nerve cells.

When alcohol makes its way to the brain it affects judgment and reasoning, then if you continue drinking it diffuses into other parts of the brain affecting speech and vision, with the next drink your blood alcohol continues to rise affecting voluntary muscular control, causing you to stagger and slur your speech. At this point respiration and heart action is compromised and the drinker's brain center becomes completely overwhelmed and subdued, and they pass out—"thank God for little favors". Any higher dose gives the body an anesthetic effect that could stop breath and heart. Large amounts of alcohol consumption can lead to the accumulation of ammonia, which is toxic to the brain. This is why you hear about young college kids dying at a party from alcohol; they drank so fast that the effects of alcohol continued to accelerate after the person had gone to sleep. Party a lot, drink ample alcohol, get a buzz from another substance, take an antidepressant, and then go home. You realize you need sleep right away so you take a sleep med or Tylenol PM with another drink. In the case of Heath Ledger, there was immediate speculation he had overdosed on illicit drugs, but autopsy reports ruled this death an accidental toxic combination of prescription painkillers, anti-anxiety medication, and sleeping pills.

ALCOHOL and BODY WEIGHT

Alcohol should be looked at as eating a high fat snack or dessert because your metabolism interactions occur between the macronutrient fat and alcohol in the body. In that alcohol receives preferential treatment, which means when presented with both fat and alcohol, the body stores the comparatively harmless fat and disposes itself of the toxic alcohol by burning it off as "jet" fuel at the rate of 1 ounce in 1 hour. Having a mere 3 oz. of alcohol reduces fat burning by about a third which when combined with a high fat diet can promote fat storage particularly in the central abdominal area. Let's face it no matter "how" we rationalize our drinking habits, it interferes with our digestive process and metabolism. Other factors that enter into this double-crossing fat storing beverage are genetics, type of diet, gender, exercise, and other lifestyle habits.

Alcohol provides your body 7 calories per 1 gram and fat provides 9 calories per 1 gram and 28 grams equals 1 ounce. Therefore alcohol consumption on top of a person's normal caloric consumption of food is fattening both through the amount of calories it delivers and through its effect on fat metabolism. The reasoning is that ethanol is a much less complicated molecule, super easy to digest and absorb fast so the body simply gives it the red carpet treatment the moment you take that first sip. In fact, it gets absorbed and metabolized before most medications and nutrients. Fat just happens to be the most efficient metabolic way to pack on the pounds. On the other hand you utilize a small amount of calories when your body tries to turn carbohydrates and protein meals into body fat. Regardless, any food loaded with fats whether omega-3, 6, and 9 or monounsaturated, saturated, or trans fatty acids will immediately get access to your belly, saddlebags or any other area your body directs it to be.

Typically alcohol reduces appetite—making people unaware that they are hungry. But in people, who are tense, uptight, type "A" personalities or the sick and the elderly who have lost interest in food, small doses of wine taken 20 minutes before a meal improves appetite. The key beverage here is wine. The congeners of wine are credited with this improvement. Wine in moderate doses improves morale; self-esteem, stimulates social interaction, and promotes restful sleep.

Factoid: Congeners are chemical substances other than alcohol that account for some of the physiological effects of alcoholic beverages, such as appetite, taste, and aftereffects.

The more alcohol calories you budget the less nutritional food you can eat. It doesn't stop here; alcohol abuse not only displaces nutrition from the diet but also affects tissue metabolism. The more alcohol you drink, the less likely that you will eat enough food to obtain adequate nutrition. The cell tissue's metabolism of nutrients goes haywire. The inadequate food intake and impaired nutritional absorption that accompanies alcohol abuse can lead to many vitamin deficiencies. Bottom line alcohol abuse disrupts the way your body does business.

THE HANGOVER
Myth   Mixing drinks is what gives you a hangover.
Truth   Too much alcohol in any form produces a hangover.

Remember the movie The Hangover, when Ed Helms, Zach Galifianakis, and Bradley Cooper "come to" after a crazy night of bachelor-party revelry, they find a baby in the closet and a tiger in the bathroom and they can't seem to locate their best friend Justin Bartha, the groom. After an episode of drinking your body may exhibit the similar symptoms of a hangover, which range from headache, upset stomach, and nausea, dry mouth, loss of memory and the worst, severe tremors, which requires medical management. I can't over emphasize that alcohol is a narcotic as well as a depressant, which produces the effect of a drug withdrawal. The actual hangover is caused by:

. Alcohol Abuse
. Mixing or switching drinks
. Dehydration of the brain
. The byproduct of formaldehyde in the body

The cure for a hangover is simple. Don't over indulge with alcohol, drink water between your drinks, and give yourself plenty of time to drink that drink. Remedies like vitamins, tranquilizers, aspirin, drinking more alcohol, breathing pure oxygen, exercising, and eating a particular food is useless. Fluid replacement is the only way to normalize the body's chemistry.

THE UPS AND DOWNS of ALCOHOL

The benefits associated with moderate alcohol consumption:

. Reduce your risk of developing heart disease, peripheral vascular disease and intermittent claudication

. Reduce your risk of dying from a heart attack

. Possibly reduce your risk of strokes, particularly ischemic strokes

. Lower your risk of gallstones

. Possibly reduce your risk of diabetes

The risks associated with anything over moderate to excessive alcohol consumption can lead to serious health problems:

. Cancer of the pancreas, mouth, pharynx, larynx, esophagus and liver, and breast cancer

. Pancreatitis, especially in people with high levels of triglycerides in their blood

. Sudden death in people with cardiovascular disease

. Heart muscle damage (alcoholic cardiomyopathy) leading to heart failure

. Stroke

. Blood pressure

. Brain atrophy (shrinkage)

. Cirrhosis of the liver

. Miscarriage

. Fetal alcohol syndrome in unborn child, including impaired growth injuries due to impaired motor skills

. Suicide

People with certain health problems probably shouldn't drink any alcohol. If you have:

. A history of a hemorrhagic stroke

. Liver disease

. Pancreatic disease

. Evidence of precancerous changes in the esophagus, larynx, pharynx or mouth

. Family history of alcoholism
. If you are pregnant

The following target population should avoid drinking alcoholic beverages:
. Children and adolescents.
. People of any age who cannot drink moderately.
. People who plan to drive, operate machinery, or take part in other physical activities that require focus, skill, decision-making, or coordination to maintain safety.

Myth   Alcohol is a stimulant.
Truth   Alcohol depresses the brain activity.

Alcohol reacts and interacts with many common frequently prescribed drugs and over-the-counter medications so check with your doctor and pharmacist before drinking any type of alcoholic beverage. For example, if you combine alcohol with aspirin, you increase your risk of gastrointestinal bleeding. And if you use alcohol and acetaminophen (Tylenol and other brands similar), you increase your risk of liver damage. The United States Food and Drug Administration requires all over-the-counter pain relievers and fever reducers to carry a warning label advising that those who consume three or more drinks a day to consult with their physicians before using the prescribed medication. Do you, or your family and friends take any of the following medications? If so, please note that people taking prescription or over the counter medications will have a reaction of some type when drinking alcohol. Alcohol alters the effectiveness or toxicity of many medications and some medications may increase blood alcohol levels.
. Antibiotics
. Anticoagulants
. Antidepressants
. Diabetes medications

. Antihistamines
. Anti-seizure medications
. Beta-blockers
. Pain relievers
. Sleeping pills

So if a person drinks and uses another drug at the same time, the drug will be metabolized more slowly and will exert a more potent effect. This happens because your body is busy disposing of the alcohol, so the drug cannot be handled until later; which initiates a dose build up to where its effects are greatly amplified sometimes to the tune of an overdose.

Case in point, when a heavy drinker on prescription mediations stops drinking there is no alcohol to compete with other medications, so the drugs are metabolized by the liver much faster than before, which makes it hard to determine the correct dosage of a medication that was prescribed when that individual was typically under the influence of alcohol. So it may be a good idea to visit your doctor to see if you need to change the dosage.

More on the Downside of Alcohol

Alcohol does for the drinker what nicotine does to the smoker, robbing the body of vitamins and minerals.

. Stomach cells over secrete both acid and histamine causing inflammation.

. Intestinal cells fail to absorb thiamin (required by the brain and neurological functions), foliate (required for blood formation and digestion), vitamin B6 (needed for healthy blood), and other vitamins.

. Liver cells lose efficiency in the activation of vitamin D, which alters production and excretion of bile. Liver cells experience a reduced capacity to process and use vitamin A.

. The kidney starts to excrete magnesium, calcium, potassium, and zinc,

. Rod cells in the retina, which process vitamin A alcohol (retinol) to the form needed in vision, find themselves processing drinking alcohol instead.

. Wernicke-Korsakoff syndrome characterized by paralysis of the eye muscles, poor muscle coordination, impaired memory, and damaged nerves which can be treated with B vitamin thiamin yet to recover from this chronic condition you would need to reduce or stop your alcohol intake so you could metabolize your food.

. Contributes to heart disease, stroke, and birth defects.

. Inhibits the production of new cells and the rapid dividing of cells of the intestine and blood.

. Alcoholic beverages can interfere with your ability to absorb and use calcium. And its diuretic quality promotes calcium loss through urine. Finally, alcohol may counteract any beneficial effect calcium has on blood pressure.

When we take a look at alcohol and regulation of body weight, a variety of systems exist to maintain body weight whether it be your set-point or some other predetermined point.

Studies with both animals and humans have demonstrated the real existence of controls. Your regulatory systems involving the brains neurotransmitters oversee the activity of feeding. The catecholamines, norepinephrine and dopamine (neurotransmitters made from amino acids) are then released by the sympathetic nervous system (SNS) in direct response to dietary consumption. These neurotransmitters govern the activities associated with the hypothalamus, a part of the brain that senses a variety of conditions in the blood then signal other parts of the brain or body to adjust those conditions when necessary.

Alcohol neurotransmitters affect the hypothalamus and its perception of consumption needs. There is evidence to suggest regulation takes place on both a short and long-term basis; short term regulation of body weight and consumption needs referring to factors such as hunger, appetite, and satiety; while long term regulation involves a signal from the body's adipose (fat) tissue when normal body composition is disturbed as in weight loss.

Myth　Wine and beer are mild and do not lead to addiction.
Truth　Wine and beer drinkers worldwide have the highest rates of death from alcohol-related illnesses. It's not what you drink, but how much, that makes the difference.

Calories Associated with Alcohol Consumption

Bourbon/80 proof	1.5 ounces	95 calories
Bourbon/86 proof	1.5 ounces	105 calories
Bourbon/90 proof	1.5 ounces	110 calories
Brandy/80 proof	1.5 ounces	95 calories
Brandy/86 proof	1.5 ounces	105 calories
Brandy/90 proof	1.5 ounces	110 calories
Gin/90 proof	1.5 ounces	95 calories
Gin/86 proof	1.5 ounces	105 calories
Gin/90 proof	1.5 ounces	110 calories
Rum/80 proof	1.5 ounces	95 calories
Rum/86 proof	1.5 ounces	105 calories
Rum/90 proof	1.5 ounces	110 calories
Scotch/80 proof	1.5 ounces	95 calories
Scotch/86 proof	1.5 ounces	105 calories
Scotch/90 proof	1.5 ounces	110 calories
Vodka/80 proof	1.5 ounces	95 calories
Vodka/86 proof	1.5 ounces	105 calories
Vodka/90 proof	1.5 ounces	110 calories
Whiskey/80 proof	1.5 ounces	95 calories
Whiskey/86 proof	1.5 ounces	105 calories
Whiskey/90 proof	1.5 ounces	110 calories
Beer	12 ounces	160 calories
Nonalcoholic beer	12 ounces	32 calories
Red wine	4 ounces	85 calories
White wine	4 ounces	80 calories
Margarita	4 ounces	270 calories

| Daiquiri | 4 ounces | 225 calories |
| Pina colada | 4 ounces | 262 calories |

Lite on Tap

| Amstel Light | Beck's Premier Light | Budweiser Select |
| 95 cals/5g carbs | 64 cals/3.9g carbs | 99 cals/3.1g carbs |

| Coors Light | Corona Light | Heineken Premium Light |
| 102 cals/5g carbs | 99 cals/5g carbs | 99 cals/6.8g carbs |

| Michelob Ultra | Miller Chill | Miller Lite |
| 95 cals/2.6g carbs | 110 cals/6.5g carbs | 96 cals/3.2g carbs |

| O'Douls | Sam Adams Light | |
| 65 clas/13.3g carbs | 119 cals/9.6g carbs | |

If you want to include alcohol in a calorie-controlled diet plan, then drink no more than one drink per day for women and no more than two drinks per day for men. A "drink" is defined as 12 ounces of beer, five ounces of wine or one-and-a-half ounces of 80-proof liquor. You will need to account for such beverages in your daily caloric consumption. A good strategy is drink with your meal. It keeps you from drinking too much. How alcohol effects your body weight depends on your overall diet and exercise plan.

This brief commentary is meant simply to open your mind and explore some of the ways alcohol can affect your mental and physical wellness. Alcohol is noted by the news, popular magazines and television networks as a contributor in too many deaths, disturbing and uncontrollable behaviors that are connected to our young, aging, and famous. In the case of alcohol, the most assured path to health and wellness is to refuse it altogether, but knowing the social pressure and advertising dollars put into our celebrated alcoholic beverages; if you decide to drink, do so

in mindful reflection of the potential outcomes and in moderation. Talk with your pharmacist. They will know a lot about the
substance you have been prescribed. These facts don't mean that
you can't drink moderately and maintain a healthy weight, but
rather pointing to the ugly fact that this delightful beverage is not
a diet drink. You booze you lose.

Source: U.S. Department of Agriculture, Dietary Guidelines
Advisory Committee, Nutrition and Your Health Dietary Guidelines for Americans, 5th ed., 2000, Home and Garden Bulletin no.
232, available at www.usda.gov/cnpp or call (888) 878-3256.

10

How the Heart Decides

Not All Love is Created Equal

A colleague who was writing an article regarding "Love" relationships called me up and posed the question—where, how, and when do we meet the one we're meant to be with. Was there an event or decision in one's life that created the differentiation? So I said, "What I understand you are asking is how does one make a decision and what factors influence our choices in love?" The law of attraction and the brain's neuroplasticity is a complicated subject. Love itself is linked to the universal field of intelligence that connects all things, including people and relationships that enable us to experience deep satisfaction, sadness or fulfillment or in our lives. The virtue of love itself can be traced back 3,000 thousand years to the time of Aristotle and Plato, Aquinas and Augustine, and the Koran. In Tibetan Buddhism, the samurai code, Lao-Tze, and the Old Testament and lets not forget Confucius, Talmud and an American Icon Benjamin Franklin. Of course what love meant to Benjamin Franklin differs in interpretation than that of Plato or Buddha. In order for people to make significant strides when in love, they need to experience a fundamental shift in their entire brain's thought system. This shift in ones brain requires a period of rewiring allowing the brain to reside in this state we call love. After the brain becomes rewired, less effort is needed to consistently evoke the notion "falling in love" allowing us to live the benefits of being intimately connected to the one we love or the things we love. Since the beginning of time, the idea of love has been reinforced and endorsed by most religions, and philosophical traditions. Love is even said to be the foundation of humanity and the basis of positive social interaction with others. Yet this fundamental shift in thinking occurs through our brain's ability to change its structure and function through the power of thought. Think about that for a second, your experience and encounters change your brain. As an example of modern pop culture, the idea of love became a global sensation when the Beatles on their 1967 album Magical Mystery Tour, sang the song "All You Need is Love."

Like ice cream, love comes in many flavors, the love of a child, breed of dog, friends, type of car, style of home, color, and then there is the elusive concept "falling head over heels in love." Of course, Scientists are the first to say that falling in love is much more than affection in return for the feeling of another person or object. When talking about the concept of falling in love, these emotional connections are deeply embedded in the neuropathways of our brains making the one we love seem irreplaceable to us. For decades, scientists have studied the probability and process of how we love. The scientific community tends to believe that the power of emotions stand in the way of rational thought yet without feelings there would be no need to reason. Scientists have found that while emotions can overwhelm the brain you can't be rational without being emotional, because your emotions help form and predict future thought, making love a perpetuating cycle.

The first thing I should tell you is that science has arrived at a consensus that falling head over heels in love with that special someone takes about a fifth of a second. The second most interesting bit of information was found in a new meta-analysis study conducted at Syracuse University called "Neuroimaging of Love," by Professor Stephanie Ortique. Her research concluded that the act of falling in love produced a similar response to that of using the addictive drug cocaine that affects the brain's faculty to think clearly, reason and apply knowledge or new information. In addition, the findings gave neuroscientists and mental health professionals' new insights on how falling in love or being heartbroken can cause emotional stress or depression. The real chemistry that touches the biology of love is far too complex to put into words, as science still has not validated every single possibility for the attraction between two people. All that science aside, the scope of what has been studied is how the brain processes the feelings connected to love within the mind and body. Scientific research can assure you that it is important to feel not just intellectualize about the one you love.

Your mind may rule your heart but it doesn't always do what you want. When in love the brain makes you have sleepless nights over the smallest changes of heart carrying the consequences of every neurological pattern associated with ones mind, each love struck moment, conversation and decision.

When wrestling over whether that person is the right one or wrong one the brain appears to be deceptive. When captured by love instead of tying down your emotional mind give it lots of space allowing your brain to observe the part of yourself that has ben taken over by the feelings of eternal bliss. Yeah, when it comes to passionate affection it is easy to understand that the human brain is the most complicated object in the known universe. In fact, choosing who to be with or what to do is right up there with thinking associated with airplane pilots, NFL team plays, movie directors, poker players, investors, chefs, and serial killers. The emotional state when falling in love causes our body to release a flood of feel-good euphoric inducing chemicals that trigger specific mental and physical reactions. You've been there, I've been there, and we've all had an emotional bout on the rollercoaster of love. Your heart goes pitter-patter; you get that warm flushed feeling all over your body, and you become an unconscious incompetent otherwise known as a babbling idiot. Think of the initial feelings of love as a mild, impermanent form of obsessive behavior. It really doesn't matter if you're in love, infatuated or attracted to the "right" person or the "wrong" person because in either scenario the mind and body is highly engaged with a "chemical cocktail" which overwhelms one's ability to use their brain to exercise common sense. The feeling of attraction to that particular person is like craving your favorite food becoming so powerful it can lead to long lasting happiness or problems in relationships reinforcing the notion that love is blind or at least unpredictable. While researching love, I came to the realization that the actions of falling in love were more scientific than we may have seriously thought through. A brain in an intimate relationship is like a sponge drinking up the spill of each and every moment. When falling in love, did you know the brain records every smell and taste making the pace and process of falling in love a perfect experience for all our senses. The condition of being closely tied to another by ardent affection becomes obsessed with a continuous desire to caress, kiss and spend time with that special someone absorbing every memory, assigning a meaning to everything experience from a first kiss to a favorite song. When choosing that special relationship, life partner or just accepting a date, your brain becomes completely involved on multiple levels. The factor of perception or what I refer to as an illusion or better yet mental distortion provides the human mind a thin line between a good decision and bad decision. The tenderness of strong, enthusiastic liking for another takes the form of faith or insanity. It becomes almost impossible for friends and family to persuade the brain of a love-bitten individual that they have taken leave of their senses. The notion that love is blind depicts the early stages of love, which I will equate to the honeymoon stage of relationships, idealizing the one you have chosen and only seeing the traits you want to see. Scientists and psychologists feel the brain may behave in this unseeing non-judgmental mode for a higher biological purpose. Scientists found that if judgement is delayed, the most unlikely pair could get together, survive and reproduce.

Love is in the mind of the beholder. Everyone who has ever

been in love wants to believe he or she at the time was a ratio-nal creature, but alas we are definitely not. When the brain is clear about the difference between love's reality and emotions it changes the way our brain talks to us. When we make those love decisions we suppose that we consciously analyze the al-ternatives and carefully weigh the pros and cons of intelligence, attractiveness, or humor, referred to as an exercise in decisional balance. But it turns out when in love we don't take the time to mindfully measure the positive or the negatives of the moment, in fact, a decisional balance sheet of comparative potential gains and losses don't even surface till we are knee deep in the clutches of love or worse, the breaking up stage. Daniel Amen, psychia-trist and brain disorder specialist along with other neuroscientists have discovered through MRI scans that just thinking of the one you love lights up the brain's pleasure center. It should come, as no surprise the chemical cocktail within the brain is equivalent to being drugged or intoxicated. The brain's pleasure center is com-posed of the neurotransmitter and hormone dopamine creating the feelings of euphoria along with the stress hormone adrenaline and norepinephrine that quickens the heart beat, strengthens the force of the heart's contractions while constricting the blood ves-sels, opens up the bronchioles in the lungs, and increasing blood pressure and blood glucose. Like taking a bite of your favorite food, falling in love is fast and intense creating an obsession to be with that person 24/7. This rise in neurotransmitters and hor-mones explains why this instinctual drive of humans motivates their choice in a partner. You and I know this selection process as romance, which represents specific biological cues that enable us to select a desirable mate. Of course there is no rhyme or rea-son but in todays contemporary society researchers have found that men and women spend an enormous amount of mental and physical energy with the rituals of falling in love rather than the primal process of conceiving babies.

As long as people make decisions, they will find themselves forced to think about how they made those love, life or death choices. Researchers have written elaborate theories associated with this process of love and the brain's decision-making finding there are three phases of love, which include lust (sexual arousal), attraction (romantic attraction), and attachment (emotional bonding). Lust is purely emotional and hormonal, attraction is all about your brain becoming fixated and obsessed with every detail of that person, attachment is the body developing a tolerance to the pleasure of that person creating a state of well-being and a sense of security. Every response is regulated by the brain's use of chemical cocktails.

Here is where the brain on cocktails gets a little sticky—you can be bonded with one person, excited by another and have a whirlwind night of sex with yet another person. Isn't that normal on most reality TV shows? There are many aspects of the human brain accounting for the variations in attraction cues just like our food preferences or other pleasurable habits. In fact, scientists have mapped the chemical changes that occur in the brain when in the initial stages of courtship and have seen the parts of the brain that are activated when in love and of more interest, the parts that are shut-down. What they have found is that the brain head over heels in love titters on the edge of nervous and unstable.

Like a dog with a favorite toy, ultimately it seems the human brain is no different than any other animal. Which comes down to the brain's intellect fighting against its primal emotions inside our head then using the heart to justify and rationalize the answer we want rather than what we know is really right. I repeat, like a dog with their favorite toy. Let's face it, life is much too contingent, complex, and emergent ever to conform to a formula surrounding the delights of the brain. The obstacle course for falling in and out of love is all about rupture and renewal; each decision to have a relationship defines and refines our thinking, helping to mold and create our identity.

THE FACES OF LOVE

A quote I saw from LiveLifeHappy.com stated, "The brain is the most outstanding organ. It works for 24 hours, 365 days, right from your birth until you fall in love." In modern society, the knowing-about love has vastly outpaced knowing-how to love. Reality TV programming models love in its finest with the Bachelor, The Bachelorette, the Kardashians, and other popular shows. We can find a gazillion articles and books surrounding how-to-manage just about any aspect of match making, love making, dating, flirting, keeping the romance alive, keeping sex interesting or how to make-up and break-up. As in the romantic comedy "The Break-up," starring Jennifer Aniston and Vince Vaughn, this movie reinforces the reality that love is not always a happy ever after situation. When the brain breaks-up it initiates a new mental context, which starts a detachment dialogue with itself—or instance, you may ask yourself how you got to this point. Then your brain creates a new mental script confirming that you have gone above and beyond for that person. You've cooked, picked their crap up off the floor, bought flowers and booked surprise vacations—been romantic, compassionate, and supportive. In fact, you have taken care of everything. And you just don't feel like your appreciated. In fact, you feel like they have lost their passion for you. The problem with this belief comes down to human rationality. Knowing what should be done and being able to do it are two different things. Especially in the matters of the heart, decisions are made in the excitement of the moment, coming down to a visceral reaction to a confusing and sometimes difficult decision. The brain in love, can't and does not reason; at least not very well. Losing love is never easy to understand much less talk about no matter what the reasoning may be. The country music scene has documented song after song of the plight of the heartbroken brain. It all comes down to those darn chemicals again. Scientists have found that when choosing a partner people may be attracted to particular biological cues, yet their selection of the ideal partner is composed of various factors that are not always based on chemistry but rather an exercise in contextual thinking. Studies experimenting with speed dating found that modern human mate choices followed a "like-attract" pattern, where people choose mates who matched their self-perceptions. For instance, many times we talk about how our friends feel like family. And many times this extended group of friends are actually more similar to one another than our own family members. James Fowler, a professor of medical genetics at the University of California, San Diego, who study's shared genetics, found that smell for instance was a gene that friends were more likely to have in common. This shared commonality of smell suggests that the ability to tolerate or be drawn to a certain scent may actually influence our decision on where to go and who to hang out with. Now think a moment of all your friends and how many times you've actually gotten introduced or arbitrarily meet the one you will date, love, or eventually marry at one of these shared hangouts. Genetic researchers call this the "Starbucks effect" because you're drawn to the smell of coffee where others with the same preference are attracted. And voilà you meet the one you end up marrying. You meet because you both loved coffee and you make friends because you all love coffee. Of course the Starbuck effect happens with sport, movies, restaurants or whatever you and your friends are into on a regular bases.

Love is more than a basic emotion—love also involves cognition. The brain has been studied by many scientists and is not a black box so let me give you my best take. Our brains and how we think is really a complex and messy process. Many parts of the brain are involved with the production of emotions. Whenever anyone makes a decision, the brain is full of feelings, driven by its inexplicable passions. When in love for instance, even when we try to be reasonable and restrained, these emotional impulses influence our judgement. Though we know right from wrong, this doesn't mean that our brains come preprogrammed for good decision-making. Feelings can lead us astray and cause us to make all sorts of predictable mistakes. The simple truth is that making good love decisions or any decision, requires us to use both sides of the brain. We are both rational as well as irrational. We tend to rely on statistics or the "ole gut" instinct. Researcher tells us that there are three kinds of LOVE. First is love of the person who gives you comfort, acceptance, assistance and who nurtures and bolsters your self-confidence. Second, is love of the person who depends on us for these life provisions? Third, is the idea of romantic love, idealizing another person, their strengths and virtue while conveniently downplaying their shortcomings.

THE TRUTH BE TOLD

Honestly decisions of the heart are based on your "frame of reference" an illusion created by mental distortion which is composed of past experiences combined with your five senses, personal beliefs, not-so-valid assumptions of life in a complex world. As a result natural selection gives us a brain that is enthusiastically pluralistic. Which means that reality is composed of a multiplicity of ultimate feelings and emotions. Some of the time the heart needs to consult the brain and reason through the options and carefully analyze the possibilities. The secret I think is knowing when and how to use "perceived thought." When trying to determine whether that special someone is the right one, by thinking about how we arrived at this junction. It comes down to a real time life simulation. There is a benefit in experiencing various love-hate scenarios and that comes with taking time out in the real world, exposure to a variety of situations, individuals and ages. Someone needs to develop a computer program that allows us to practice falling in love and make decisions—then cues us on developing helpful behaviors for successful relationships, similar to the phone app called Kissing Test. Scientifically, we need to understand our choices in terms of competing brain regions or the firing rate of neurons. I know by now you're thinking, OMG so cold and scientific but unfortunately this is at the heart of the matter. Knowing ourselves from the inside out can reveal many unexpected surprises.

Love is the force that bonds, unifies and makes creation possible while the power of love enables our lesser self to rediscover the better self. Love is allowing your brain to slip between the cracks of perception, of what appears as real. Then comes true love, with its preexistent unknown information unseen by the brain yet with enough power to retain the love experienced at first sight. The only real geography in love are the mental markers created by the brain's memories; it is not whom we love but rather what we have become in the process of love that makes the difference in a life. Love is a way for our brain to transform and experience one's self over and over again. Love is the standard and choice that ultimately drives the process of falling for that special someone.

First, the brain doesn't make any choices in a vacuum but rather in the context of the real world or should I say your world composed of past and present experiences. Second, we can't make any choices without emotions or emotional intelligence.

LOVE TALK

When an individual in love is drawn to a specific person, the mind is trying to tell them that he or she should choose that option. Yet, subconsciously, that individual has already unconsciously assessed the alternatives. That analysis takes place outside of the conscious awareness of the mind and converts that assessment into a positive emotion just like an obsession to eat your favorite food or purchase a pair of Jimmy Choo shoes. Each and every person has a different interpretation or flavor of what love looks and feels like making it difficult to define. The basis for the emotion itself is mysterious, begging the question why do I love this person over that person. In his book *Too Soon Old, Too Late Smart*, Gordon Livingston, M.D. asked his readers to think about this definition, "We love someone when the importance of his or her needs and desires rises to the level of our own." Then Livingston cuts to the chase and gives his reader an operational question regarding proof of love, "Would you take a bullet for that person?" He then acknowledges that of course this idea is extreme since few of us can say with certainty what we would do if our self-preservation was challenged by our love for another. The virtue of love is reflected as the manner in which we choose to behave. While the actions of love influence our brain to operate differently, narrowing our focus towards the one we desire. Let's take a moment to discuss ones capacity to love and to be loved by another.

. If you find it relatively easy to get close to others, and you feel comfortable depending on them and having them depend on you. And don't often feel worried about being left out and abandoned, or getting too close then you have secure love.

. If you feel somewhat uncomfortable being close to others, feel your partner wants more intimacy than you are comfortable giving, find it difficult to trust them completely and allow yourself to depend on them or get nervous when they get too close then you have avoidant love.

. If you find yourself being reluctant to get close to others, worry that that person doesn't really love you or won't want to commit to a relationship or merge completely with you than you have an anxious love.

THE WINDY ROAD OF LOVE

I am not sure if you can really sway the outcome of the heart to love or not to love. To think we can capture the love of someone strikes me as more of a hopeful fiction movie with Meg Ryan that we all cling to in such heart filled situations. Real honest to GOD love doesn't afford us the luxury of caring or not caring but rather affirms the act of caring. The process of "how" we fell in love can reveal itself slowly, the gradual accretion of all the seemingly mundane every day acts of being responsible, kind, and compromising in the face of adversity. True unconditional love is stripped of all its bells and whistles. The process of love itself creates baggage and emotional damage that accrues overtime, forgiven yet never forgotten. Many have lost the "look of love," a connection between saying "I love you" and understanding the real meaning of it. Most individuals simply adopt a scientifically removed state towards love to insulate themselves from love's pain and uncertainties. As a result, they become emotionally stunted, less likely to care about relationships. Falling in love is an amazing process, yet the commitment of love is defined by inevitable heartbreak built on decades shared with the person you are likely going to see die.

LOVES SHAPES AND SIZES

Love comes in numerous shapes and sizes. When you find yourself in love, the thinking-brain connection is severed, like a computer with a virus; we can't comprehend our own emotions because we have lost access to the brain's wealth of opinions that we normally rely on for those choices. All of a sudden you no longer know what to think about that person. It becomes very confusing as to what is a good idea. The end result is that it becomes impossible to make a decent decision. What will they like, where should we go, how should you look, dress, and talk, comes down to a Las Vegas crapshoot. The thinking process has been disrupted, our reasoning smashed apart. Love is like a daytime soap opera. A new episode is filmed every single day. Think about it, everything feels sincere, even when what is happening on screen is completely crazy. When it comes to love just enjoy the moment and when it doesn't feel right, don't try to make it work by making sense. That is just nonsense. The silver lining is that everybody possesses a wellspring of love, renewable at any time, allowing us to be sensitive to impressions, desire, and the emotional state of love. The brain in love sees the possibilities, develops a broader way of thinking, allowing you to transform your life for the better by building your resources and strengths. As the seeds of love grow, our brain flourishes with new possibilities, the capacity to be remarkably more resilient and content with our circumstances in life.

THE SUCCESSFUL HEART

Tolerating the complexity of love is probably the greatest challenge of the mind; requiring the same effort as it takes to balance oneself on a bicycle. In 1989 Psychology professor Bob Levenson, a UC Berkeley professor discovered that loving couples that made it to "death do us part," instead of divorce, worked at problem solving and compromise. His researcher then uncovered another interesting twist—it was the wives not husbands that calmed marital conflicts, which strengthened the couple's chances of staying together. Levenson found that couples developed appreciative understanding for each other's values and ideas, taking pride in their partners' accomplishments, and no longer attempted to change one another but rather exercised acceptance. 78 pairs of fortysomething married 15-plus years and 78 pairs of sixtysomething married 30 years concluded that couples have plenty of problems, conflicts, and unforeseen difficulty yet in a loving committed relationship these couples learned to work through the day-to-day challenges. Researchers believe the reason most of these couples made it to the 15-year mark was their ability and willingness to resolve life's problems together. It came down to the spouse being a safe harbor and best friend. The study determined that wives were the key, not the husbands when it came down to de-escalation of a heated argument. If the wife could calm down shortly after the conflict, the marriage had a better chance of succeeding. And the husband's ability to regulate his own emotions had little to no role in long-term marital satisfaction. Now that is a brain reframe if I ever heard one. In today's world of DNA testing researchers have discovered a connection between relationship satisfaction and gene variant. It turns out you and I inherit the gene variant from our parents. Couples in the studies were found to be unhappier in a marriage that was full of negative emotion, like anger and contempt, or a short mental fuse. On the other hand, happy couples displayed more moments of good emotion, including laughter, humor and affection. Happy or unhappy you have to be careful in drawing any vast conclusions around DNA, genetics and marriage. But you must admit that this research does introduce a whole new wrinkle into the understanding of relationships of the heart.

In excavating the brain, how you love someone may hold few clues about your potential relationship. Like all thought provoking decisions some people are predisposed to being happy or unhappy, judgmental or non-judgmental, skinny or overweight. Just like being on a diet, managing your weight starts with the mental attitude of eating healthy and working out, and will lead to good health. What seems to ring true about the well-shaped and happy relationships is that they just keep connecting, good or bad, for better or for worse, conflicts or celebration, and just work at it. Understanding the biological cues and necessities behind the process of love gives insight into the complexity between instincts and impulses. To uncover your full capacity for love, consider your life as a whole. Think about each and every time your brain felt in love? What were the triggers that set love in motion and what nourished its growth? What were you doing at the time? Viewing love in this way can sharpen your capacity to see love as a momentary state rather than a word that defines a relationship between two people. There is no one answer, rule of thumb, generalization, consensus, or magic potion that allows love between two people to flourish. Humans send and respond to all sorts of biological cues from one another and these cues can trigger feelings and attraction. Yet it is a brain imperative to understand what works for you because scientists have repeatedly found that love is highly individualized, reflecting a sense of our current circumstances. How your brain falls in love might be completely invisible to family, friends and the general public yet everybody's capacity to give love or be loved by another may differ greatly, which means your path to discovery will be unique. These intimate relationships could best be seen as the movie "Groundhogs Day" starring Bill Murray and Andie Mac-Dowell or "Edge of Tomorrow" with Tom Cruise and Emily Blunt as the products of recurrent surges of love. Words of advice—

love, learn then love again. Whether looking for a commitment, simply dating or deciding to have an affair, when falling in love don't drown yourself in words and emotions, because we are not what we think, feel or say but rather what we do.

11

The Perpetuating Cycle of Stress

Problems = Stress and Stress = Problems

Though exercise is a proven stress reliever, there are three other vital components of managing stress – situation, perception, and reaction. Exercise may relieve tension and anxiety, promoting focus and concentration yet it doesn't target the causes of stress. Without altering your situation or your perception of the situation, whether it is school, work, relationships, or health problems, stress will continue to rear its ugly head. To reduce stress and improve your mental and physical health, learn to break the stress cycle through management of the situations, how you perceive the situations and your reactions to the situation.

Daily mental stress starts in the brain yet many times those stressors are expressed through the body, manifesting in numerous ways mentally and physically. In fact, there is significant and convincing scientific evidence that stress, positive or negative, can contribute to a broad array of health related issues that contribute to added difficulty, uncertainty, and perplexity. "Between 60-90 percent of the complaints brought to a doctor's office are due to stress," claims Dr. Herbert Benson, president of the Mind/Body Medical Institute at Harvard Medical School. It seems that all forms of pain – mental or physical – can be made worse by a person's mental health, state of mind, or degree of stress. Managing the cycle of stress requires an individual to shift their energy (emotions), redirect focus (mind) and resurrect an enhanced self (body). It is all about getting in shape mentally and physically. Research and studies surrounding the stress factor point out that the link between physical health and mental wellbeing cannot be ignored. The mental and physical aspects of an individual must be treated as one integrated unit. To live a low stress, active and healthier life, you must be able adjust to the world and people around you, allowing maximum effectiveness and sense of happiness. You must possess the ability to habitually rethink life's problems in such a way as to derive a feeling of "can do" and personal satisfaction.

Positive or negative stress should be viewed simply as a disruption in one's expectations turning off and on in varying degrees from a passing thought, to anxiety, upset stomach, feelings of depression, constant exhaustion, headaches, weight gain, and painful periods, just to mention a few. The key is to stop focusing your mental energy on what you expect to see. Even relatively short periods of mental stress may cause unwanted changes in your life that leave brain cells hypersensitive for weeks. Instead of trying to predict the outcome of a specific circumstance why not refocus your thinking on the strategy that could be employed to make, do, or accomplish the task at hand. The brain can take on the challenge of change when new expectations are generated that allows the achievement of something desired, planned or attempted. Once the mental energy begins to flow the mind and body can work as a unit again. The key to managing stress is mental health or a "state of mind" permitting the optimal exercise of one's talents and the steady movement toward satisfying one's needs. Mental health is not an all or nothing proposition but rather an exercise of relative magnitude. Degrees of mental health vary from person to person and day to day.

Life experiences lend to perception and interpretation of reality, affecting one's stress and overall mental health.

TYPES OF STRESS

There are two types of stress: distress, which produces negative effects such as anxiety leading to tension, pressure, pain, lack of focus, and poor performance, and eustress, which produces a positive effect such as anxiety leading to motivation and accomplishment. Exercise is classified as eustress. Whether positive or negative, acute or chronic, stress needs to be managed.

Distress initiates chemical changes in the brain, stimulating the release of neurotransmitters, such as serotonin, epinephrine, nor epinephrine, and acetylcholine. These chemicals act as a stress communication system in the body. In response to this to this complex communication network (neurotransmitters), the heart rate, blood glucose production, and blood pressure may increase.

Eustress of exercise boosts the production of the body's natural pain relievers and mood modulators known as endorphins. Endorphins are thought to cause a euphoric feeling in the body, like morphine, and counter the effects of distress.

Although exercise tends to relieve stress and anxiety, it can also perpetuate stress. The psychological stress caused by competition is an obvious stress producer. Less obvious, yet equally important, is the emotional stress experienced by a working woman determined to integrate an exercise routine into her daily schedule. The process of trying to coordinate all of her activities into one day can create considerable emotional stress and anxiety. The point being, the mind and the body must be treated as on unit. The psychological factors may be more important than we realized and may contribute to a variety of dysfunctions within the body.

Define your stressors
. Chemical
. Physical
. Emotional
. Neurological
. Environmental

. Technological
. Nutritional

THE BRAIN'S PLIABILITY AND CAPABILITY

A resilient mindset is what allows an individual to manage and change beliefs, behaviors and assumptions. It seems the management of stress and accompanying mood disturbances may be one of the key factors that influence your resilience. With a resilient brain serving as the focal point, an individual can influence their thinking, better absorb stress, and skillfully plan for the future. Resilient thinkers possess the pliability and the capacity to rebound after a stressful event faster, allowing them to sidestep the quagmire of dysfunction, rather than becoming a victim of stress. The resilient thinker faces the same challenges as everyone else when confronting stressful situation. Yet they regain their equilibrium faster, maintain physical and mental health while achieving a higher level of mental performance and productivity. It is not that a resilient thinker is less susceptible to life's stressors nor that it can prevent the disruptive effects of stress, but rather the flexible mindset allows the brain to bounce back quickly. The resilient mind has the capability to create, accept, and rehearse new thinking. When confronted with the fast-moving, high-stress conditions of rapid cognition, how suited a person's decision may be to their end purpose becomes a function of ability, willingness and practice. The resilient thinker comes from the mindset that no suggestion can be denied. The right frame of mind and framework all of a sudden engage the brain in a fluid, effortless dialogue of creative thinking.

THE DEMANDS OF STRESS

The stress process is initiated when a chemical, physical, emotional, and/or neurological demand is made on an individual. Demands fall into two categories—those that are self-generated or externally imposed at home, work, or within the environment. Self-generated demands are driven by self-imposed standards.

What is truly "real", "valid", or "relevant" in any given situation is a matter of opinion, which means "how" and "what" your mind perceives, interprets, and react to can vary depending on your state of mind. This statement validates the importance of your "Frame of Reference" (FOR) and its influence over mental stress. Stress should be viewed as an aggregate coming from such sources as the workplace, problems at home, lack of stress, commuting from home to work, a major life event or intense interpersonal exchanges, substance abuse, over medicating, poor nutrition, chemical imbalance, and physically over-training or under-training just to mention a few.

The way in which our brain's perceives and interprets a request, demand or potential threat will determine whether or not a stress reaction occurs. Each and every person on this planet sees life through different lenses. This is why there are extreme differences in how people react to the same stress stimuli. Perception dictates how that individual will interpret and in turn react to a stressor. And that thinking forms our expectations and determines how we process the information, which allows alternative decision making and what actions are taken.

When facing a new danger or opportunity, write down every strategy, approach or solution to the problem. When you force yourself to write down your thoughts, you increase the chances of having new insights that can sway your perspective and instincts. Your beliefs, behaviors, and assumptions of a person or situation serves as a mental map or guide to what actions you consider appropriate or inappropriate when engaging life. Ones level of mental stress reflects how strongly that individual holds true to these guideposts.

Beliefs—the consistent set of integrated values and expectations acquired over time that provide the framework for shaping what an individual believes true or false, relevant, good or bad about themselves, the environment and the world around them. How far you drift from your belief system determines the level of stress response and reaction.

Behaviors—these are the observable interactions the brain has recorded that constitute "how" and "what" an individual does day to day. And those behaviors reflect how close the interaction aligns to the individual's expectation.

Assumptions—represents the unconscious rationale for continuing to apply the same logic, belief or specific behavior to a given situation. Individuals tend to develop patterns of behavior, based on the outcome. For the sake of efficiency your brain relies on these familiar patterns of behavior whenever confronted with a similar circumstance. Eventually, the uses of these patterns become part of the individual's automatic unconscious decision-making process.

Whether positive or negative in nature, all of us react to stress to some degree. Stress is merely a reaction to how you interrupt a perceived reality or threat. When stress reaches out and grabs your mind it teaches you a lot about rapid cognition referring to the brains unconscious automatic ability to find patterns in situations and past behaviors based on a very narrow slice of experiences. Yet this type of decision-making is elusive and deceptive. How is it possible to gather the necessary information for a worldly-wise judgement in such a brief moment? When on autopilot the mind's stress effect is put into motion by a set of involuntary psychological and physiological changes called the "fight or flight" response. It is the very same response that helps an animal get ready for conflict or to escape harm. The mind and body taps into its stored energy, transferring it from fat cells and the liver to the muscles. Then the body enters into a survival mode. This survival mode affects people on psychological, behavioral and physiological levels. For example, psychologically, a person may seem irritable, anxious, unfocused and short sighted. Behaviorally, some symptoms are restlessness, tremors, loss of sleep, and problems speaking. Physiological symptoms are those associated with "fight or flight" include shock, surprise or alarm, which could result in elevated blood pressure, increased heart rate and other physical responses.

But here is the kicker—there is a large body of evidence suggesting that stress-related diseases emerge because we activate a physiological system that has evolved for responding to occasional physical emergencies. Our brains are turned on for months on end, worrying about whether or not we have a job, get a promotion, keep up the appearance, pay down the stack of bills, pay the mortgage, juggle the kids, and care for elderly parents. Living a high voltage stressful existence 24/7 without recovery will simply kill you.

A prominent lawyer friend of mine once taught me a valuable lesson regarding overreacting to any given seemingly stressful situation. He taught me that everything that happens to you in life doesn't necessarily require immediate attention. And if you can learn to wait a while, the situation, decisions and individuals can actually resolve themselves with time, conserving a lot more mental energy. Over time I found he was right! If we live in a continuum of stress, we must train ourselves to spin each and every event into an opportunity for learning. For example, if you're laid off your job, see it as an opportunity for a new beginning or shift in your career. I am not asking you to be OK with being laid off, especially if you have a wife and kids, a school loan and bills, or other demands. But to simply stress out won't do much more than make you sick, tired, and relationship poor.

Studies surrounding happiness have shown that people who aspire to have fame, fortune and the perfect life are less happy than those who learn to engage in daily activities they find fulfilling and pleasurable. Money can't buy you happiness or a stress free existence. Despite the fact that over the past thirty years we have become richer as a nation, studies suggest we have as much if not more stress than in the past. We have become a nation of technologically stressed overachievers. If we want to maximize the brain's effectiveness we have to learn to manage the stressors in order to conserve mental energy. This is especially true in today's time-crunching life, with so much time being devoted to work and the "pursuit of happiness" and not enough time being given to the business of leisure, recreation, nutrition, exercise, and recovery.

COPING WITH STRESS

When the only tool you have in your tool kit is a hammer, you tend to treat everything you experience as a nail. Coping with stress is more like the transition of an ice cube that is melting, eventually becoming liquid and refreezing again when the circumstances are right. There are volumes of research aimed at coping with stress, associated behaviors and stress reduction techniques. Handling stress means controlling the noise in your head and getting a handle on your mental activity. In truth, no event, no person, no one situation can give you permission to "stress out." What triggers stress is solely your response to what you and your brain see as a stressful situation. You have the capability to revisit and rewrite that mental interpretation. When you contemplate something stressful, real or imagined, you prime the body to fend off actual physical danger. Unless you find ways to interrupt this mind-body feedback loop, your stress level will sustain and self-perpetuate. It comes down to what you think about and how you assess an event that determines your response.

Managing your perception of life is probably the most important aspect of stress reduction. If you can shift your frame of reference or see the situation in a different light, you may feel less threatened and gain a sense of control over your emotions. Ask yourself; is your perception or assessment of the situation really accurate or could you be over dramatic? Or are you over-thinking and simply reading too much in between the lines. Then evaluate your expectations, giving yourself permission not to be upset because it is just not worth it. Martin E.P. Seligman, Ph.D. and author of Authentic Happiness says that objective good health is barely related to happiness; what matters is our subjective perception of how healthy we are and it is a tribute to our ability to adapt to adversity that we are able to find ways to appraise our health positively even when we are quite sick. Whatever your circumstance, you have the ability to choose your reaction. You have the power to assign meaning to your life. In the words of Dr. Phil McGraw, one of the foremost experts in the field of human functioning, "There is no reality, only perception." How you interpret the circumstance is entirely up to you.

Emotional stress leads to physical reactions and there are no two ways about it. Just recall the pit in your stomach or the tightness in your throat or the pounding in your head when you heard bad news, or the butterflies you felt just before an important presentation or first date. Physical responses to extreme bouts of stress can lead to serious consequences such as high blood pressure, elevated risk of heart attack or stroke, weight gain, suppressed immune system, irritated bowel syndrome (IBS), sexual dysfunction, ulcers, migraines and insomnia. For example, my ability to sit through a Martin Scorsese film, war movies or any movie where humans are threatened with extreme violence causes my heart rate to quicken, my adrenaline to surge and emotional distress. I actually want to leave the theater.

We work so hard to maintain a healthy mind and body. Preventing stress has turned into a management issue. The development and implementation of stress management skills enables a person to avoid some stress-evoking situations, thereby evading the wear and tear that accompanies stressful episodes. Become more accountable for your response to stress and the problems in your life. Revisit and test your belief system by maintaining an active, ongoing awareness of your response to situations, and recognize how you could have avoided or altered your behavior. You always have the choice of whether an event will be your undoing or a constructive learning. In the words of Eckhart Tolle, author of *Power of Now*, *"There is no past there is only the now."* The past is over and the future hasn't been written yet. The only time is now.

Effective strategies to combat stress include:
. Revisit your belief systems and change your response
. Challenge, reprogram, and change your thinking
. Stop being overly sensitive
. Get learning out of every situation
. Take a problem-solving approach
. Maintain a balanced diet
. Get enough sleep and recovery time
. Listen to music
. Monitor caffeine, alcohol and drug abuse
. Take up a hobby
. Increase your physical activity
. Communicate with friends and family
. Limit your technological communication
. Prioritize and trim back your commitments
. Practice deep breathing techniques, relaxation, and meditation

Meditation can bring balance to your life by clearing the noise in your head and help to find inner space. When we perform a relaxation technique, we're stimulating activity in the parasympathetic nervous system, which is the same system responsible for slowing your heart rate and relaxing certain muscles. Such activities can offset the effect of the body's overly activated stress response including blood pressure and rate of breath when practiced on a regular basis.

The successful acquisition and application of stress management techniques must be transferable and generalized. To increase transferability and generalized stress management techniques, you should practice coping skills (in the form of new behaviors) in situations that are identified to evoke stress. Repeated performances reinforce the strength of the new behavior while incorporating the new response into the new behavior repertoire. For example, if you are dieting, most people have been told, "if you do not buy it, you will not eat it." I think this is solid advice yet why can't you buy it and practice eating your favorite food in moderation? Another example we have been taught is to avoid individuals who stress you out, but why can't you learn how to deal with difficult people? Life demands flexibility and change—and change brings disruption and stress. Stress associated with life change can build great learning. Life isn't fair or perfect so learn how to navigate your mind and manage your life.

STRESS CHECK

Stress is not the enemy in our lives. Stress is a normal physiological response of the body when faced with a hostile situation or environment. Stress affects everything and everyone and paradoxically it is the critical factor for mental and physical growth. Though the stress factor may be different in different age groups, the outcome is more or less the same. The effects of stress on the body can be categorized into short term and long-term effects irrespective of the age groups.

When the trigger is repetitive, prolonged or unanticipated, then it becomes pathological. The immediate, transient or short-term effects are the normal physiological responses, whereas the delayed, persisting or the long-term effects of stress are the pathological responses.

The Canadian endocrinologist Hans Selye originally introduced the notion of stress in 1978, generalized as a physiological reaction that came about when the body was exposed to any kind of extraordinary demand. After a bout of stress, Selye discovered we foster the development of energy far beyond our normal run of the mill needs and limits physically, environmentally or emotionally. Whether the stressor is physical or psychological, coping skills are required to eventually help that individual overcome disruption or insult to their mental and physical system. Generally speaking, research indicates that information helps the individual with expectation setting while the factor of time allows for adequate mental and physical preparation.

A reaction to stress takes three forms: emotional, behavioral and physiological. These factors are typically experienced together in various degrees depending on the individual's personality characteristics, nature of the stress, and the emotional reaction to the stress. When you are presented with a stressor positive or negative in nature, regardless of the cause, your body produces neuropeptides that exert a negative effect on the brain triggered by the production of the hormone cortisol, which in turn can affect your health when produced in large amounts. More stress produces greater the amounts of cortisol production.

The effects of stress on the mind, heart, respiratory tract and nervous system have been well studied and documented. Medical sciences are working on ways to help individuals understand and manage their response to stressors. Stress disrupts your ability to effectively manage life's complexity while draining you of assimilation capacity. This silent killer has the ability to attack the body on many levels.

These are the effects of stress on your mind and body:

Brain – lowers the production of disease-fighting blood cells, which in turn contributes to depression, agitation, anxiety, and insomnia and in some cases, short-term memory loss.

Face – stress induced over stimulation of hormones, can create lines around the mouth, blemishes on the skin and other effects including dry mouth, jaw clenching and other skin disorders.

Hair – excessive hair loss and some forms of baldness; stress has no effect on hair color.

Eyes – strain, dark under eye circles, temporary blindness and conjunctivitis.

Reproductive Organs – menstrual disorders, recurrent vaginal infections in women, inability to become pregnant; impotence and premature ejaculation in men.

Digestive Tract – can cause or aggravate gastritis, stomach and duodenal ulcers, colitis and irritable colon.

Heart – major contributor to cardiovascular disease and hypertension.

Chest – shortness of breath.

Neck and Shoulders – promotes the release of chemicals into the nervous system that speeds up muscle deterioration.

Back – pain and muscle twitches.

Hands – sweaty palms and tremors.

Source: The American Institute of Stress, John Hopkins University School of Medicine and National Institutes of Mental Health.

EFFECTS OF SHORT TERM STRESS

Any form of stress that elicits a strong emotional or physical response has the potential to expand our capacity for change. Hans Selye maintained that a body reacts to stressors with a nonspecific sequence of processes that he called the *general adaptation syndrome (GAS)*. When an individual encounters a threat, Selye theorized that the body gets prepared to handle the situation by means of 'Fight or flight' response. The initiation of a stressor unleashed certain functional adjustments within the body. Resources are activated by such physiological changes as increased rate of heartbeat and resperspiration, dilation of pupils, a drop in body temperature, increased perspiration, and release of glucose into the bloodstream. When the threat no longer exists, the body returns to normal. These immediate, transient effects are the short-term effects of stress. This is a physiological response seen in all individuals exposed to stress. The few functional adjustments, which are responsible for the short-term effects, are:

. Diversion of the blood from less vital to more vital organs.

. Increase in the heart rate to supply more blood quickly.

. Increase in the blood pressure to supply blood efficiently.

. Increase in the respiratory rate to get more oxygen from the atmosphere.

. Breakdown of glycogen stores in liver and muscle to get more glucose.

. Formation of more glucose from non-carbohydrate substances.

These functional adjustments responsible for the stress effects on the body, manifest themselves with an array of signs and symptoms which include:

. Palpitation
. Chest pain
. Frozen shoulder
. Cold clammy skin with gooseflesh
. Flushing and feeling of warmth
. Breathlessness
. Dry mouth with difficulty in speaking and swallowing
. Abdominal discomfort
. Aggravation of Peptic Ulcer
. Loose stools
. Increased blood glucose levels.
. Headache, back ache and neck pain
. Depletion of physical and mental energy
. Flare up of diseases like eczema, psoriasis, arthritis
. Difficulty in concentrating
. Memory disturbances
. Sleeplessness
. Decreased sexual drive
. Loss of appetite
. Anxiety
. Depression
. Outbursts of anger

EFFECTS OF LONG TERM STRESS

If the stress persists and becomes repetitive, the body keeps secreting the stress hormone cortisol. Here more intense, longer-acting defensive measures are put in place. The body now experiences stress with an extra burden due to the side effects of the persistently high stress hormones. This can cause some irreversible physiological damage to the brain and related physical symptoms. The manifestations could be:

. Chronic head ache
. Mood swings
. Anxiety disorder
. Substance abuse
. Memory disturbances
. Heart attack due increased blood pressure, sugar and cholesterol
. Stroke due to similar reasons
. Weight loss
. Exacerbation of allergies including asthma
. Irritable Bowel Syndrome (IBS)
. Ischemic Bowel disease (IBD)
. Decreased sexual drive
. Sleeplessness

Even when the stress factor is absent some of these physical and physiological effects of stress persist unless steps are taken to treat them.

POST TRAUMATIC STRESS DISORDER

Post traumatic stress disorder (PTSD) is a delayed reaction to an exceptionally stressful situation or a life-threatening event where the person feels helpless. After a dormant period the person re-experiences the past traumatic events as 'flash backs' or dreams, and tries to avoid any stimuli or situation which reminds them of the past trauma. The symptoms include:

. Psychological numbing
. Amnesia of certain aspects of the stressful event
. Inability to experience pleasure
. Isolation

. Reduced interest in activities
. Sleeplessness
. Agitation

You may be asking yourself if managing mental and physiological stress worth the extra work? All evidence indicates that the management of stress probably won't guarantee fame or fortune but rather assist in managing the mindset that shifts ideas that hold intrinsic value in the future. When wrangling with stress, like a doctor faced with a tough laborious diagnosis, challenge your mind's uncertainty by asking yourself for a second opinion. But be warned whether your thinking is based on first impressions or cautious deliberation, the brain's instincts can betray us. Instead, learning to manage and question your level of stress will bring new definition to "what" and "how" you decide to operate in the world and in turn lead to more control over life satisfaction. Your new found sense of awareness will help even out the genetic differences that may have disrupted your thinking giving you a new perspective on reality. Whether presented with high or low stress, our brains have more or less the same structural makeup. How you interrupt the stress is what makes the difference in brain activation. It comes down to learning, which creates connections between neurons, and fluctuations in neurotransmitters, the chemicals that surge through the brain. One of the most critical components to stress reduction is learning to be present and aware of the moment. Making sense of our behaviors and our selves requires first impressions as well as rational analysis. With new learning comes the added benefit of understanding. A healthy brain is needed to improve your chances for survival in a continuously changing and uncertain world. The demand and challenge of brain change is the ultimate reason to manage daily stressors. Who knows what you may face in the future? You are now fluent in stress management with an understanding that only a healthy brain can produce a unique and innovative future and life satisfaction.

12

The Brain's Control Over Change Intelligence

How Intelligence Correlates to an
Individual's Brain Capacity

In the words of Zoe Weil, cofounder & president of The Institute for Humane Education and author of the book, *Most Good, Least Harm*, "Living your epitaph may be the most important ingredient for inner peace and serenity. In other words, when you actively align your choices with your life's purpose and goals, you live more honestly, more courageously, and with greater integrity, and these virtues bring with them a powerful kind of freedom". But how do you retrain the brain and develop change intelligence? It becomes less a matter of perspiration than of cultivation and nourishment to keep growing new connections in the brain. Brain change evolves while toiling in the fertile soil of our own lifescape where fresh associations produce new thinking. Of course, psychologists refers to general intelligence based on five factors that are tied to IQ:

Crystallized intelligence acquired through knowledge and skills gained through experiences, formal and informal education or training.

Fluid intelligence reflects our in the moment reasoning and problem solving ability, not dependent on background knowledge, education or any specific expertise. Being a fluid thinker allows us to identify connections and relationships when in new situations.

Visual-spatial intelligence combines the ability to visualize, remember and manipulate images in the brain. Visual processing is measured by tasks that require the placement of objects as they move through space. Processing speed requires a high level of attention and focused concentration and is a measure of how fast your mind processes information. Processing speed is your ability to automatically and fluently perform basic cognitive tasks like scanning a paragraph for a specific phrase or word.

Short term/working memory holds in mind a limited amount of information for a brief period like remembering a cell phone number or recalling the directions to a location. It is called the working memory because it gives you the ability to mentally transform information, to figure something out, or reason through a problem. The more short-term memory you develop the more processing power you possess.

Quantitative intelligence is based on an individual's store of mathematical knowledge and well-practiced techniques for solving mathematical and quantitative problems. The brain's intelligence correlates to an individual's capacity to entertain original ideas, make new connections then applying that unfamiliar thinking within a new context. Like the unquestioning quality of faith, the joining together of new ideas is inevitably constrained by the state of mental acceptance of something even though absolute certainty may be absent.

Maintaining an open, flexible mind starts to question and breakdown the brains firmly held perceptions and ossified habits, assembling a new order of thought by rubbing away old thinking. Steven Johnson author of *Where Good Ideas Come From* believes we take the ideas we've inherited or that we've stumbled across in life then we jiggle them around in our mind to reshape a new way of thinking. Yet until new learning occurs, there are doors that cannot be unlocked. Brain change is a story of one door leading to another door and to yet another door, giving us an opportunity to explore and learn one room at a time. In the words of Niccolo Machiavelli, "One change always leaves the way open for the establishment of other." The course of continuously developing ones brain occurs through a shift in thinking that allows that individual to explore the edges of new possibilities that surround them. Being programmable or receptive to new ideas means your life becomes "open-ended", allowing you to more easily question beliefs, behaviors or assumptions to accommodate new needs. David McClelland, Research Professor of Psychology and author of Human Motivation, correlates that animals and humans share factors of change intelligence in his research surrounding what variables and in what combinations would best predict responses and how often and how strongly it would be made. McClelland went on to point out environmental situations were obvious precursors. He then references motivation by stating the obvious: a hungry rat will run faster through a maze or learn the correct turns more quickly than a satiated rat, but only if there is food in the goal box and only if the rat can get into the maze.

McClelleand supports the fact that change does not happen through good intention rather there must be a driving force, a need that must be filled. If you can change your way of thinking, you can change the world you live in. Some individuals find change intriguing and respond with enthusiasm. Others find change disruptive and unpredictable, interfering with the day to day of getting things done. Even the most mentally flexible person can't resist certain types of change due to volume, complexity, and time constraints. Exceeding your change tolerance activates the human instinct to seek stability, familiarity and control of what happens. Yet reinventing yourself is not as easy as simply trying new life strategies, you have to implement the right change decision at a point in time where it can be more easily understood, accepted, and internalized. Most of the time the mind's old belief systems block and limit new thinking, obscuring new opportunities from being considered due to the factor of "uncertainty," making the current state so mentally uncomfortable that you justify the status quo and discard the need to change altogether. In today's contemporary high tech environment it is not enough to just react to events. To make the most of each situation mental intelligence dictates we should establish a conscious objective from which we can select our actions to get nearer to what we need.

The process of intelligent reasoning enacts the need for a sound objective put into place with the best possible actions that produce the desired effect. The conscious intelligent thinker goes one step further by observing results, learning and storing the experience for an alternative plan of action for future circumstances. Intelligence itself is defined as a general set of cognitive problem-solving skills. Change intelligence is what you do when you don't know what to do. The capability to acquire change intelligence starts by allowing your brain to shaking free from past good or bad experiences.

"There is nothing permanent except change." Heraclitus (540- 475 B. C.). Change intelligence is defined by the brain's current established patterns and habits. The brain change process is affected by your ability to predict the desired outcome: expectations cloud your perception, which influence your comfort level and what you're willing to shift, which sways thinking and alters which actions are taken. The most important precondition to change intelligence is to be capable of adopting new ideas. By definition a rigid mind sets up a self-fulfilling prophecy, incapable of forming new patterns of thinking making it impossible to probe new ideas. What initiates the change process is the myriad of connections that unfold with the introduction of new experiences. The brain assimilates new information then assesses strategies for responding to a change decision or situation. The challenge is "how" to create a new environment that fosters new thinking that allows new connections in your personal life, within the workplace, and across society itself. You can't use the power of the mind, conceive ideas, draw inferences and make judgments without practice. Intellectual skills can only be cultivated through effort. Most individuals view their intelligence as a fixed unchangeable mindset, they strive to obtain positive evaluations of their ability and discount evidence of inadequate ability or unfamiliar information. The unconscious intelligence is demonstrated in task performance by the notion they either have or lack ability. This negative self-concept influences the acceptance of new information, applied effort and observed learning. The views your brain adopts for yourself profoundly affects the way you lead your life and determines whether you become the person you want to be. The brain involved in the transition phase of change behaves differently, finding value in new behavioral shifts that start to reshape the thought process. The changing brain pays close attention to information that could stretch their knowledge. Additional factors that tamper with ones capacity to retrain ones brain deals with the volume or number of decisions, specific timelines, require re-education, learning and new skills. The message to those wanting to enhance intelligence is not to take on more brain changes than you can assimilate. Christopher G. Langton a computer scientist and author of *Artificial Life: An Overview (Complex Adaptive System)*, 1997, observed that innovative systems have a tendency to gravitate toward the edges of chaos which is equivalent to thought that vacillates between too much control and anarchy.

The concept of synergistic thinking $1 + 1 > 2$ is the only option allowing the complexity of information to produce a greater effect than working in a vacuum. Synergistic thinking engages the mind's capability to interact between factual and conceptual information producing a new and deeper understand similar to that of working with others to generate more ideas and solutions while consuming less mental energy. In order to grow ones thinking during the transition process you must be willing to live with some inner tension on a personal, professional, and environmental level. Mental fitness requires viewing lifestyle change as a continuum not an event. Research shows that the brain is more like a muscle-the more you use it the stronger it gets, the more synaptic connections, and the more the brain cells multiply and grown. Retraining the brain is affected by how we organize the facts to be heard, encoded and decoded and only at the conceptual level do we have the transfer of knowledge and intelligence.

Life nowadays is fast paced, bringing with each day a new twist or turn. Everything you see, read, and hear dictates another set of changes you should be considering from the fashion pages of Vogue, to the newest diet craze, future financial investment, next level of health care considerations, and don't forget global warming. Continuous and overlapping change has become a way of life—accelerating, voluminous, and complex.

While most individuals focused on compiling fitness assessment and developing a functional exercise program the value for retraining the brain is left unattended. Most individuals treat lifestyle change and behavior modification as an event rather than a constant state of flux, from birth until death. Optimizing your ability to successfully accept, implement, and sustain a significant behavioral shift is not only an exercise in point of view but of dealing with questioning the ground you walk on. The single most important ingredient when taking on life is becoming capable to reinvent and retain your thinking. Becoming a flexible open-ended thinker will give your mind the opportunity to not just survive shifts in behavior but to actually bounce back stronger from an unexpected setback or turn of events. Like an essential nutrient, becoming mentally flexible is the essential component that transforms the neuropathways required to retrain the brain. It is what distinguishes those individuals who achieve behavioral change versus losers who achieve only temporary superficial change.

13

The Brain and Its Habits
The Preprogramming of Autopilot

Immanuel Kant, a German philosopher considered a central figure of modern philosophy believed that the human ability to create concepts from our view of the world, its laws, and reason was the source of our morality. Little did Kant realize he was the first to actual identify what we call today as habits, a settled or regular tendency or practice, especially one that is hard to give up. Also referred to as custom, routine, pattern, way, norm, tradition, rule, or a matter of course. Many psychologists consider habits as the brains way of learning from our day-to-day encounters. In fact, there are volumes of books dedicated to the best of human habits. *The 7 Habits of Highly Effective People: Powerful Lessons in Personal Change* by Stephen R. Covey or *The Habits of Being Yourself: How to Lose Your Mind and Create a New One* by Joe Dispenza. But as you know life can be too decisive, determined by someone or something else, complex, and unexpected to conform to a formula. And then there is the truism that knowing what one should do and being willing and able to do it are two sometimes drastically opposed ideas.

Everyone's journey has it's own blueprint but one thing is for certain, within each lifescape comes habits. Habits seem to fall into two categories, the habits that we are not ashamed to admit to like eating healthy and regular exercise, and then there are the unwanted unhealthy habits we tend to defend or avoid answering completely. When conceptualizing a habit, think of your body as an aircraft and the brain as the cockpit and within the cockpit a control panel. A habit, in essence is likened to your body being on autopilot. The preprogramming of autopilot can be compared to the brain being prewired to perform the every-day maneuvers of daily life with or without its actual involve-ment. These ingrained patterns of behavior allow us to live a lot of our lives in this mode of operation. Most of us live life running almost fully on autopilot. By this I mean that we function almost completely without thinking. Each day, you wake up, shower, shave, brush your teeth, comb your hair, have breakfast, get in your car, and manage to get to work without too much thought. In fact, most times you can't seem to get through the daily grind without routines while other days you could curse your inabil-ity to break from those same laborious, sometimes tiresome ac-tions. The power of habits is that they insure that you use as little conscious energy as possible, leaving yourself free to focus your available energy in new ways.

When changing a behavior we must choose what matters most. We must face the fact that knowing and learning opens one up to uncertainty and the embarrassment of incompetence, making us more vulnerable, making change a continual dance of learning within ourselves and from others. The view that I want you to explore is that the brain's memory of past experiences are what create your future habits. Psychologists believe that by the time we hit our mid-30's our personality is completely formed; the brain's subconscious responses and perceptions are already running our lives. In fact, researchers think that 5 percent of the mind is conscious, struggling against the 95 percent that is sub-consciously running your brain's day-to-day programming. In other words, the operating system of your subconscious mind acts as a computer program behind the scenes of your conscious awareness. How could this happen to your brain without your knowledge of it? Well, neuroscience has a principle called Hebb's Law that simply states that nerve cells that fire together, wire together. This idea demonstrates that if your brain repeatedly activates the same nerve cells, eventually those stored thoughts and patterns of behavior will develop a long-term relationship called a mental signature. And this mental signature becomes your signature personality. The combination of thinking the same thoughts combined with acting the same way, and feeling the same emotions, begin to enrich these patterns of behavior. Mahatma Gandhi simple said, "Your beliefs become your thoughts, your thoughts become your worlds, your words become your actions, your actions become your habits."

The brain's thought processes create habits for everything you do, which in turn controls what you think, feel, how you learn, remember, move and talk. The brain has been referred to as the organ of personality, character, and intelligence. The issue with habits is that the brain processes both the positive and negative habituations in the same way. And like any muscle in the human body, the more your brain experiences a particular pattern of behavior, the stronger those habitual patterns good or bad become. Whether it's overuse of technology, overeating, over training, learning a language, or driving your car, researchers are of the opinion that all patterns of ingrained behavior become habits and are based on the same types of brain mechanisms. This brain-intensive process referred to as creating habits, rituals, behaviors, or adaptations, is an indestructible neurological fact of life. The bad news by Joe Dispenza, the author of many books surrounding the brain once said, "The greatest habit you could ever break is the habit of being yourself." To reinforce Dispenza's notion of habits, Albert Einstein once stated that no problems could be solved from the same level of consciousness that created it. Einstein believed if you wanted to change habitual patterns and attain this new state of "being you," you must create a mental picture regarding how you must act, how you must think, how you will talk, walk, feel all the way down to your look. The key to changing unwanted habits is not knowledge, but rather the understanding how to apply that knowledge. If you want to outsmart your unwanted tendencies, you need to think smarter. It sounds like a simple fix, however, when the brain is on autopilot, the operating system becomes susceptible to quick fixes and mindless behavior as it bumps up against unforeseen situations or the newness of a circumstance.

When attempting to break free from these unwanted ingrained patterns of behavior, what must be kept in the forefront of the thinking brain is what needs changed and how will that thinking help you navigate through the process of restructuring your unwanted habit. But according to Daryl Conner, a thought leader in the field of industrial psychology and author of *Managing at the Speed of Change,* "People tend to discount new information that is inconsistent with their current beliefs and patterns of behavior." Conner's research found the secret to changing all habits lies in shifting one's perception of reality. These perceptions of reality could be compared to a protective membrane; allowing you to absorb the repercussions of life; insulating the brain from the disruption of having to change those inclinations. Think of it this way, your reality represents a mental landscape of those habits that have positively effected you in past life experiences. These preferred trusted behaviors have been nurtured many times over a lifetime. The brain's belief system tends to tightly cling to those habits or patterns of thinking which allow it to get through today and the unforeseen future. The problem starts here, if you keep thinking the same thoughts, do and feel the same things, you're basically hardwiring your habits into finite patterns that reflect your finite reality. You know sometimes a crash landing becomes necessary to promote the vital restructuring necessary to transform the thought process of the thinking brain.

Yes this newness is uncomfortable in many ways because it represents unfamiliar territory. But when confronting a habitual change in behavior, the only option you have is to take steps to strengthen an alternative behavior by creating a new neurological web of connections or suppress the original habit, which will weaken the previous neurological pathways that exist in your brain.

When it comes to patterns of behavior, I personally have fought many battles yet have never lost site of the war. The key to breaking old habits emphasizes a basic principle of training referred to as the Training Effect. Improvement or creating a Training Effect refers to the physiological changes that occur in the mind and body as a result of sufficiently applying the factors of frequency, intensity, and duration to exercise. This principle applies to all types of physical and mental demands. Whether you are breaking or forming a habit or becoming proficient at an exercise, the more you do it, the easier it gets. The longer your brain continues to practice the activity, your mind and body starts to adapt and a learning effect gets downloaded to the brain which in turn gives your mind and body the training effect.

The components of breaking unwanted habits can be achieved when you:

1
REPLACE – Replace those unwanted habits with alternative competitive actions. In other words, substitute an interesting new activity for an unwanted behavior as a powerful way to create a new positive behavior. Become aware of the triggers that make you vulnerable to unwanted habits. This requires your thought process to be receptive to new possibilities that challenge and compete with those old practices. The caveat to replacing the unwanted habits comes down to planning; the alternative action must be available and able to be performed at a moment's notice. And the alternative activity must be appealing enough to compete with the unwanted behavior.

2
CONQUER – Conquer your unwanted habits. Unwanted behaviors are triggered only at certain impulse moments. These brief periods of time push your brain to forget any alternative action

and it is at this point in time you break your positive momentum by potentially giving in to the urge of an unwanted practice. The impulse moment is a critical tipping point in the brain's conscious attempt to conquer the unwanted habit, because of the potential to derail even the best attempt to change.

3
RELINQUSIH CONTROL – If you want to transform your mind you must lose your objective mind and let go of the perceptions of your current state of reality. You must give up the old mindset of what you think you know and become fully cognizant of the unconscious patterns of behavior you wish to change. With consistent practice, redirecting your urges starts to build new patterns on which to create your new self. Disengaging from the habit of being yourself contributes consciously and energetically to making room for the new you. To make it over the finish line, you need to have carved out an alternative appealing strategy, one that can compete with the negative power of your unwanted behavior.

4
REPETITION – A signature personality required lots of practice and rehearsal time. Repetition helps form the neurological web of patterns that will become familiar to the new you. Feed your brain with new knowledge, experiences and learning, allowing your neurons to weave new connections. The more your brain cells fire together the easier to produce the new thinking at will. Like an amazing actor you must think, act, feel and become that character. This is when you are ready to go on stage.

The only justification for changing ones behavior is to enhance a person's capacity to produce a desired outcome. As Ralph Waldo Emerson said, "That which we persist in doing becomes easier—not that the nature of the task has changed, but our ability to do it has increased." Achieving specific results requires behaving in a way that produces the desired result. In other words, you and your habits are the ones held accountable for defining, shaping, redirecting and living your life in a mindful way. All you need to do is step up to the plate with new thinking, inspiring ideas, and a willingness to experiment, rehearse, learn from mistakes and retry all over again. The body, mind, and energy all exert an influence in actively shaping future behavior and you either consciously take them into account or stand back and watch the damage unfold. "The best way to do is to be," said Lao Tzu about 2,500 years ago. And in the words of Clark Terry, an American Wing and bebop trumpeter, "Keep on keeping on."

14

The Recovery Process
Mind and Body Performance

ONE BRAIN ONE BODY

Dr. Robert Ward, author, coach, player, elite athlete, professor, and scientist, once said, "The mind and body are one unit, and therefore, they should not be thought of and physically trained as separate parts." When addressing Ward's concept of mind and body connection, it becomes important to wrap his words around behaviors that enhance performance. The elements that can influence the efficiency of the mind and body although difficult to predict, are factors and traits that provide the framework of interactions that take place between the mental and physical aspects of performance. A critical component for efficiencies of the mind and body are recovery, relaxation, and sleep. Many times we waste our mental and physical capacity due to the lack of recovery so sometimes you just have to shut off the lights. Those "eureka" moments don't happen unless we build in some good ole recuperation.

The recovery process is essential to reclaiming mental and physical resources, which increases one's "assimilation capacity." And assimilation capacity is what helps us manage our lives and recover from our normal to many times chaotic day-to-day schedules. Simply put, the more assimilation capacity you have available, the faster and more effective you become mentally and physically at living life. In practical terms the amount of reclaimed energy depends on the quantity and quality of sleep and degree of intermittent recovery during the day as well as other factors such as nutrition and fitness level.

The idea, of course, is to strike the right balance between living life to the fullness and recovery. The sleep factor for instance is just something we try to fit into our lives but really don't have time for when in actuality it is during sleep we resolve many problems and have some of our best brainstorming sessions. Most people lack adequate recovery, displaying dysfunctional behavior such as lower morale, poor decision making, increased error rate or accidents, chronic tardiness, depression, physical weakness, and suicide. The cumulative effect of today's life never really gives our mind and body a window of opportunity to adequately apply its healing capacity. We survive on minimal sleep, power drinks, energy bars, and poor nutrition, as we end the day with alcohol and sleep aids. Most of us are just trying to get by, while the impacts of life's demands accelerate in volume, momentum, and complexity with no time-outs and lights on 24/7. The lack of adequate sleep depletes our assimilation resources giving way to a "healing deficit". The quality of your recovery directly affects the quality of your waking life, including your mental sharpness, productivity, emotional balance, creativity, physical vitality, and even your weight. According to many experts, sleep is the most important source of recovery in one's life and every individual is uniquely engineered to accommodate sleep needs by age, gender, and genetic predisposition.

There are many scientists that believe there is no standard number of hours for sleep. There are people who wake up well rested after seven to nine hours of sleep and there are also those individuals who feel refreshed only after four hours of sleep every night. Some scientists report that it is not a matter of how many hours a person sleeps but the quality of sleep and the regularity of sleeping habits that are important. Let's agree on the premise that individuals differ in terms of the length, timing, structure of their sleep and that each individual expresses sleep deprivation differently. To that point, Gerard Kerkhof and Hans Van Dongen, researchers in the area of human sleep and cognition have consistently found that some individuals are just more vulnerable to becoming sleep deprived than others. Research shows that individuals who are deprived of sleep for a long period of time may be more stressed and tend to display illogical behavior and mood swings. Insufficient sleep can make you irritable and is linked to poor behavior and trouble with relationships, especially among children and teens. There are even studies linking criminal behavior to stress caused by lack of sleep. Research has shown even small amounts of sleep deprivation significantly impacts every aspect of our lives from the mental expression of memory, concentration, mood and reasoning to physical performance characteristics of reaction time, muscular strength and endurance, balance, coordination and cardiovascular capacity.

We need sleep to think clearly, react quickly, and create memories. In fact, the pathways in the brain that help us learn and remember are very active when we sleep. Research has clearly shown that individuals who are taught mentally challenging tasks did better after a good night's sleep. In addition, during sleep, your body produces valuable hormones. Deep sleep triggers more release of growth hormone which fuels growth, helps build muscle mass and repair cells and tissues in children and adults while other hormones increase during the sleep cycle to fight various infections. This could be an explanation for why a good night's sleep helps keep you from getting sick and helps you recover when you do get sick.

It is well documented that sleep deprivation is a leading factor in the thousands of traffic accidents attributed to sleepy drivers every year. Then there are numerous studies associated with global disasters such as Chernobyl, Exxon Valdez, Bhopal, Three Mile Island, scientific endeavors – Challenger space shuttle in 1986, and day-to-day casualties associated with evening shift workers. Some professionals in health care, security and transportation, and let's not forget air traffic control require working at night, and in those fields, the effect of acute sleep deprivation on performance is crucial. Skimping on sleep has its price, individuals who tend to stretch their days, end up compromising their nightly sleep, becoming chronicallysleep deprived.

Cutting back by even 1 hour can make it tough to focus the next day and can slow your response time.

The neuroscience surrounding sleep deprivation helps researchers to study the relationship between the brain and behavior by observing "how" a person's behavior shifts as the brain starts to shut down from lack of recovery. By taking images of the brain showing where activity is located it is possible to correlate the behavior exhibited by an individual's brain patterns. Just as a person cannot jog for three continuous days, a person's brain cannot operate without rest or breaks. Since different regions of the brain rest during different stages of the sleep cycle, sleep cannot be cut short. In fact, if the brain does not receive a break it will soon begin to shut down for periods of micro sleep, a period of sleep lasting no more than a few seconds up to a minute. It often occurs as a result of sleep deprivation or mental fatigue. This is essentially several seconds of actual sleep that impairs cognitive function. Without adequate spaces of recovery, ones life is just a blur of doing, living, and moving.

Myth 1: Getting just 1 hour less sleep per night won't effect your daytime functioning. You may not be noticeably sleepy during the day. But even slightly less sleep can affect your ability to think properly and respond quickly, and compromise your cardiovascular health, energy balance, and ability to fight infections.

Myth 2: Your body adjusts quickly to different sleep schedules. Most people can reset their biological clock, but only by appropriately timed cues—and even then, by 1–2 hours per day at best. Consequently, it can take more than a week to adjust after traveling across several time zones or switching to the night shift.

Myth 3: Extra sleep at night can cure you of problems with excessive daytime fatigue. Not only is the quantity of sleep important but also the *quality* of sleep. Some people sleep 8 or 9 hours a night but don't feel well rested when they wake up because the quality of their sleep is poor.

Myth 4: You can make up for lost sleep during the week by sleeping more on the weekends. Although this sleeping pattern will help relieve part of a sleep debt, it will not completely make up for the lack of sleep. Furthermore, sleeping later on the weekends can affect your biological clock so that it is much harder to go to sleep at the right time on Sunday nights and get up early on Monday mornings.

Source: Adapted from Your Guide to Healthy Sleep – The National Institutes of Health.

15

Sleep Loss and Your Brain

The New Normal

How much sleep did you get last night? If you are like many individuals, you probably average six hours or less. Then there are those who actually fall asleep but can't stay asleep. This group of individuals falls into the category called sleep deprived or an insomniac. Truth be told, insomnia is Not a Normal Part of Aging but in today's fast paced society insomnia is a common complaint among all sectors of the population from young children and teenagers to the middle aged and the older adults. And it seems that the older adults in particular make the assumption that aging means no longer sleeping well. Researchers on the other hand recognize that illness, inactivity, poor sleep habits, and the inappropriate use of alcohol, caffeine and tobacco—rather than age—are the major culprits associated with this escalating problem. Fortunately, proper medical care and changes in sleep habits can often promote a good night's sleep, without the need for sleeping pills.

In the case of the older adult, a lack of exercise, an unstructured daily schedule, combined with fewer responsibilities may leave an older person at an increased risk for insomnia. Added to these risk factors are illnesses such as heart and lung diseases, depression, dementia, and chronic pain, which are common among older adults.

Why and How We Sleep

To understand the current treatments available for sleep disorders, it is helpful to know why and how we sleep. Like healthy nutrition and daily activity, sleep is important for maintaining and restoring physical and mental health, affecting both the body and mind. Fact, 17 hours of wakefulness is equivalent to having a blood alcohol level of 0.05-enough to be considered legally drunk. The authors of Sleep and Dreaming: Scientific Advances and Reconsiderations found that sleep and dreaming are necessary for recovery, learning, memory, and to regulate body functions such as blood pressure, blood sugar, and immune system. And in the book The Secret World of Sleep the author Penelope A. Lewis depicts the cycle of sleep and awakening as a process controlled by an internal biological clock located at the base of the brain. The clock can be adjusted by exposure to daylight and the pattern of daily activity. The clock is set by nature to promote some sleepiness for a few hours early in the afternoon and more strongly from midnight to 7 a.m. The sleep phase of the "sleep/wake cycle" is divided into:

. Dreaming or rapid eye movement sleep
. Shallow or light sleep, and
. Deep or restorative sleep

The stages of sleep change from infancy into adulthood with progressively less time spent in deep sleep and dreaming and more time in shallow sleep. In addition, as we get older more adults tend to be "early birds," early-to-bed, early-to-rise rather than "night owls" that go to bed late and get up late. Researchers have found when it comes to age-related change in sleep habits, most occur in the early and mid years of life, changing little in old age."

SLEEP FOR THE GROUP 60+

One measure of sleep quality is sleep efficiency, which is the amount of time asleep compared to the amount of time spent in bed. The Geriatric Mental Health Foundation points out that sleep efficiency is the only measure of sleep quality that changes significantly for those age 60 and older, and declines gradually at a rate of about 3 percent per decade. Overall, the sleep quality of healthy older adults remains relatively constant unless there is an illness. Another validated fact of aging is that nearly 40 percent of sleeping pills are prescribed to older adults, although they make up less than 20 percent of overall population. With sleep medication comes the risks of impaired memory, awareness, ability to focus one's attention, accidents, and dependency associated with some sleep pills. This makes diagnosing sleep problems in an older person much more of a challenge because of the interplay between the factors of age, relationships, physical and mental illness, and the increase in medications.

THE CAUSES AND EFFECTS OF INSOMNIA

The National Sleep Foundations views sleep problems as the cause, effect, or complication of illnesses, mental disorders, and accidents. Just like temperature, pulse, and respiration; sleep and recovery should be considered a vital sign of health. The quality of one's sleep and wakefulness can be a sign of health or illness.

The National Institute of Health (NIH) thinks of insomnia as sleeplessness that cannot be blamed on mental disorders, physical illness, medications or simple problems with scheduling. The American Board of Sleep Medicine and other sleep driven organizations believe many times insomnia can promote excessive daytime drowsiness called primary hypersomnia, which is associated with nighttime periodic leg movements, restless legs syndrome, sleep apnea, and snoring. In any case, to qualify as a sleep disorder, symptoms must interfere with social or intellectual function and occur three nights per week for at least a month. Obsessive worry about the lack or quality of sleep and the use of alcohol or sedatives to promote sleep may be both a cause and effect of insomnia. An occasional sleep problem can become persistent by self-defeating solutions and self-medicating such as spending too much time in bed, abandoning a regular schedule of sleep and waking, or using alcohol as a sleep aid.

A few days of insomnia or poor sleep can be the result of a common cold or a change in routine, like staying in a hotel. However, insomnia lasting four weeks or longer likely has a more complex cause. Any individual with insomnia that lasts four weeks or longer should consult a physician. When you talk with your physician, be sure to tell them how long you have had problems sleeping. The length of time you have experienced these symptoms is important both for diagnosis and treatment, which is why you should keep a sleep journal. Also, tell your doctor about your sleep habits and any medications, illnesses or recent events that may have contributed to your change in sleep. To find out what's sabotaging your slumber, the toll it takes on your wellbeing, and what you can do to log in more quality sleep time, check out the following snoozing stats:

Napping
Power Naps or general napping, more than often; disrupt a good night's sleep. If you must nap, take one short nap of about an hour in the early afternoon before 3 p.m. If you can eliminate naps altogether, you may sleep better at night.

Amount of Sleep
At night, limit your time in bed to 7-8 hours to ensure that sleep is continuous rather than broken up over a longer period of time. A person who tries to make up for poor sleep with extra time in bed will instead experience more awakenings and disruptions in the natural sleep pattern. By limiting your time in bed to 7-8 hours nightly, you may increase the quality of your sleep and improve your daytime wellbeing and alertness. "You can't pull an all-nighter and still learn effectively," says Matthew Walker,

Ph.D., a sleep scientist at the University of California, Berkeley. Lack of zzzzz's affects a part of the brain called the hippocampus which is key in the creation of memories.

Sleep Schedule

Like daily exercise or good nutritional habits; as you introduce new sleep habits, follow them every day of the week. An important element in getting good sleep is sticking to a schedule. So even if you have not had a restful sleep, get out of bed at the same time every morning. This helps the "sleep clock" at the base of your brain function better. There is a 40% decrease in your ability to remember information when you haven't had a full night's sleep. "Exposure to light is one of the main environmental cues for creating regular sleep-wake pattern," say Ivy Cheung, a doctoral candidate at Northwestern University. To enhance your shut-eye, schedule time-outs during the day hours to increase your daylight exposure. Researcher found morning light to be most important for the regulation of the circadian rhythms.

Relaxation

By trying different strategies, you can positively affect sleep habits that may lead to falling asleep more easily. Through daily practice of relaxation techniques, you become more aware of your mind and body and learn to recognize and reduce muscle tension.

By practicing relaxation methods consistently, you can improve your natural relaxation response. There are a variety of techniques for those who seek sleep. One method encourages the individual to progressively tense then relax muscle groups in a step-by-step manner from head to toe, then they are instructed to reflect on the feeling as tension is released. Other relaxation techniques to combat insomnia can be found in a New Harbinger Self Help Workbook called *The Relaxation & Stress Reduction Workbook* by Martha David, Elizabeth Robbins Eshelman, and Matthew McKay. These authors provide powerful relaxation techniques from a variety of proven treatment methods, including progressive relation, autogenics, self-hypnosis, visualization, and mindfulness and acceptance therapy. Education about sleep and changes in sleep habits are helpful for most persons with sleep problems. However, other treatments may be needed for those who cannot maintain good sleep habits or who rely on sleeping pills, sedative/hypnotics.

Medications

Medication may be necessary for individuals whose insomnia is not helped through changes in sleep habits and therapy and for those individuals who experience periodic limb movements or restless legs syndrome. As a first step, the individual should withdraw from stimulant beverages (like coffee and tea) and over-the-counter medications that interfere with either the quality of sleep or the performance of routine activities during the day, such as driving. Always check with your doctor first before starting, changing, combining or stopping any over the counter or prescribed medication.

. Common over-the-counter medications that impair sleep include:
   . Pain relievers (analgesics) with caffeine
   . Some cough and cold medicines
   . Decongestants with phenylpropanolamine or pseudo-ephedrine

Persons with sleep disorders should not use over-the-counter medications that are marketed as sleep aides or "PM" pain relievers (analgesics) that contain the antihistamines diphenhydramine or doxylamine. In older people, these may cause side effects, such as mental confusion or bladder or bowel disturbances.

The Food and Drug Administration (FDA) do not regulate the use of natural products such as Melatonin used as a "natural" sedative. Melatonin varies considerably in content from one brand to the next, and there is little research to support its use. For persons wishing to use an herbal product, teas made from German chamomile (Matricaria recutita) or passion flower (Passiflora incarnata) or capsules of valerian (Valeriana officinalis) are popular. However the FDA does not regulate herbal remedies and they may vary considerably in content from one brand to the next. Patients should understand that sleeping pills are a temporary solution and should be reduced and then stopped after two to three weeks under a doctor's care. Changes in sleep habits offer the best chance of long-term improvements in sleep but require the most effort.

Cognitive Behavioral Therapy

Gregg D. Jacobs author of *Say Good Night to Insomnia,* has developed a six week drug free program based on cognitive behavioral therapy combines elements of positive sleep habit change in a structured format and offers long-term benefits. Cognitive behavioral therapy and changes in sleep habits can lead to a gradual reduction in the use of sleeping pills. This approach is typically more successful than simply trying to cut down on pills without professional help. With therapy, the individual and provider work on identifying and managing situations and habits that disrupt sleep in order to establish a better, more regular sleep/wake cycle. By establishing daily routines, the quality of sleep can improve for many older adults.

You're Never Too Old to Get a Good Night's Sleep

Problems with getting a good night's sleep are common among older adults. But sleep quality can be improved with simple steps. This involves learning about sleep; practicing good sleep habits, and stopping bad habits. Treatment for sleep disorders may also include reducing or stopping medications that interrupt sleep, treating disorders like depression that directly affect sleep, and, in some cases, properly using sleeping pills.

A doctor providing help for a sleep disorder may discuss

your individual sleep habits often called "sleep hygiene" and needs, and suggest changes in your habits and in your environment. First, know what to avoid. You can try many of these sleep strategies to promote better sleep by reducing those things that make you too alert. The following can help sleep:

. Make sure the bedroom is quiet, restful and comfortable
. 7AM is prime time when it comes to exercise if you want a good night sleep and your blood pressure may lower up to 10 percent through out the day and 25 percent by night fall
. Use the bed only for sleep and intimacy, not for snacking, listening to radio, or watching television
. Go to bed and wake up at the same time each day
. Develop a get-to-sleep ritual that will let you relax before bedtime
. Avoid exercising within 4 hours of bedtime
. Avoid caffeine and/or cigarettes for at least 4 hours before bedtime
. Avoid alcohol for at least 2 hours before bedtime, and do not use alcohol as a sleep aid
. Try wearing socks to bed; this lowers your core temperature and promotes sleep
. Avoid being too hungry or too full at bedtime
. Avoid drinking large amounts of fluid after 6 pm
. Get regular exercise and daily exposure to outdoor light
. Take a hot bath 90 minutes before bedtime
. Ask your doctor when you should take medications for your heart, blood pressure, breathing or pain for improved sleep.

16

The Conclusion

Your Brain All Wrapped Up

My hope is that this book has answered three questions I'm asked most often by clients, patients, and practitioners.

1. How does my brain interfere with behavioral change?

2. What can I do to alter my thinking for successful shifts in behavior?

3. How long will it take to change my behavior?

The information provided in GOOD BRAIN BAD BRAIN YOUR BRAIN is based on observational and validated research. As a Wellness Coach and Physical Trainer with the focus in cognitive behavioral change and its management I can say with absolute certainty that the process of mental transformation is too complex to lend itself to rigid steps, so my suggestions are descriptive rather than prescriptive, based on industry practices from personal training to neuroscience. There are no fixed rules when managing uniquely engineered behaviors.

The acquisition of brain balance infers that no part of your thinking is greatly out of proportion; but this sense of balance is all-important as long as it feeds your carefully crafted belief system. Rethinking the ground you walk on is a unique blend of psychological, physiological and environmental possibilities combined with the challenges of constraints.

The numbers of variants these challenges hatch make it unthinkable to apply a set order brought about by cause. To achieve alterations in one's thinking is an extremely complex task making fixed steps unrealistic. But the more we question who we are the more we understand who we mean to be and the more pleasing a future we will craft. The condition of each circumstance being unlike or dissimilar is of value because brain change is an unfolding thought process occurring on many levels simultaneously. To achieve this moving target called mental transformation and life satisfaction, you've got to start with a flexible blueprint. You can't simply check your brain in the mirror, yet it can be guided and influenced. And although the change outcome accompanying mental transformation can't be rendered certain for quality, longevity, or success, the possibility to increase the odds are significant especially with a design in hand. You can take control of your thinking by consciously correcting those inborn behavioral patterns and tendencies when you take the time to create a mental blueprint. This plan represents the mindset needed to lay out a compelling vision; allowing you to consciously think through the necessary decisions and strategies to tackle behavioral change.

The factors affecting mental transformation are lack of exercise, poor eating habits, smoking, alcohol, excessive stress and too much technological interaction; a recipe of ingredients that lead to a deconditioned flabby brain.

According to research these life style choices will hamper your memory, problem solving skills, mood, communication skills, and brain volume as well as overall connectivity. When making up for loss or damaged health and wellness, behavioral shifts comes from taking the time to think about the changes you don't want to think about and question the information that disrupts your entrenched beliefs, behaviors and assumptions of life. When you don't prioritize your health and wellness you initiate the checking-out process by censoring the brain, which contradicts and resists our perceptions for a healthy life. How you think about the future is especially serious business when it affects your expectations, which influence perceptions, which influences the process, which influences your decisions, and which affects preferred behaviors. The quality of brain change can be directly tied to your commitment to become someone different. This means you should apply strategies that work for you and ignore the rest because there are no hard-and-fast rules. But be sober, substantive brain change comes through individual trials and correction combined with readiness, ability and willingness. My hope is that this book heightens your awareness, and expedites your learning curve so you get where you want to go sooner and with less pain and suffering.

There will be no clear line separating easy questions from hard ones. It may take months of practice and reworking the brain and it's thinking to sell you on the idea of permanent changes. This book will allow you to stack the cards in your favor. I have been down this rocky road many, many times.

Retraining the brain for a new beginning is the most exciting and validating experience I know. Don't be so married to your old patterns of thought that you fail to consider new information that might change your life forever. One thing is certain – change happens either way, so deal with the uncertainty by taking ownership over the process, allowing you to become mentally flexible and able to entertain new ideas. This happens when you willingly embrace the brain's rhetoric as consistent. Pretend that life's uncertainty has been erased and start to make confident decisions that ignore all evidence of your old beliefs. Continually remind yourself that decision can be undone or re-contracted due to unforeseen events and it will all be ok.

The people who will survive and grow out of the need for brain change will be presented with abundant opportunities. If you only take one thing away from this book remember that whenever you make a decision, it doesn't matter what your choosing between, what matters is what your brain is thinking and how you apply that knowledge. The best way to use the brain properly is to be present and aware of your mental arguments. The messy business of thinking is necessary because it helps us stay clear of our own ignorance. The mind is full of flaws, which can be outsmarted through the practice of mindful awareness; the commitment to avoid past mishaps can be side stepped allowing each one of us to become a student of our own mental circus and learn from our past performances. Your brain can always be improved at any age unless dementia or other brain disease sets in.

There is an aviation saying used in crew resource management (CRM), "See it, say it, and fix it." CRM techniques can be applied to other arenas, so why not your brain? CRM training can help broaden your brain's range of knowledge, skills, and attitudes including communication, situational awareness, problem solving, decision making, and working with others. CRM capability provides your brain a new way of thinking which makes optimum use of all available resources—equipment, procedures and people to promote the desired outcome and enhancing efficiency. A CRM expert named Todd Bishop developed a simple five step assertive statement, when handling any crisis, which I have taken the liberty to adapt to a 5-step plan to retrain the brain.

1. Be clear about what you want to accomplish. Expose your thinking to new perspectives. Question your beliefs, behaviors, and assumptions in life. Ask yourself "what" do you believe and "how" did you get that information.

2. Decommission old thinking. Analyze the situation directly and emotionally identifying "what" you are trying to achieve and "how" you will achieve the change.

3. State the problem as you see it using validated information and factual statements. What are the benefits and consequences associated with the problem to be solved? State the options that will remedy the problem.

4. Obtain an internal intrinsic buy-in and commit to the change initiative as well as seeking external support from others.

5. Be prepared to seize the moment and live to do it all over again.

Start to think about what you could do differently so that you can retrain the brain's thought process and its neuropathways. The hardest part of mental transformation is that there's no beginning and no end but rather a chronic continuum of interminable stressors day-in and day-out. The way in which our brain possesses the future tells us more about ourselves and about what we fear most in the process. Retraining the brain makes thinking more sober and life more visible. When playing life's game it is important to realize you can lose, while keeping in mind whatever happens you will experience the joy of learning. In Fred Kofman's book *Conscious Business,* he talks about the larger purpose of any competitive activity is not to succeed but rather to use the experience as a way to self-actualize and achieve self-transcendence. He goes on to say, "We discover who we are and our values through our behaviors and our dealings with other people and the world."

THE TENANTS OF BRAIN CHANGE

Assess, build and secure the necessary brain capacity to do, experience, or understand something. Critical brain performance is linked to outcomes. The brain's capability is the expression or expertise an individual needs in order to perform core life functions. Working through each day is one of the greatest challenges affecting daily life. Brain change reflects ones readiness, ability and willingness not only to engage change but also to bounce back from the behavior or act that is intentionally provocative.

Preserve your brain's assimilation capacity. This mental energy is the fundamental currency needed to retrain the brain. Your brain's capacity to think is affected by every thought, emotion, or activity. Preservation of the brain's mental capacity is accomplished when new thinking allows success in a new environment. The amount of assimilation resources we accrue determines the brain's capacity to address daily decisions, and the more resources we possess the faster our brain's can recover from the unexpected. Don't over commit to change. Trying to implement too many change strategies too fast can lead to high stress and low success. The cognitive psychologist George A. Miller published one of the most highly cited papers in psychology in 1956. He argued the number of objects an average human can hold in working memory is the magical number of 7, plus or minus two.

Overloading the brain's assimilation capacity can create a diminished or accrued effect when encountering family, friends, work or reflecting on world events. The optimal energy for brain performance comes from a balance of physical, nutritional and emotional factors. Managing ones assimilation capacity instead of time is the key to brain stress and high performance. Mental energy or assimilation capacity is measured in terms of volume of change, positive or negative perception of the change, the need for speed or timely change and the complexity of the change demand. The better our brains become at entertaining information that invalidates the established beliefs, behaviors and assumptions while accepting alternative patterns of behavior, the more mental energy we preserve.

When rethinking your thinking, sometimes the only way out of a chaotic mess is to come up with a creative alterative solution. The brain resists newness and the unknown aspects of life. The mental energy needed to assimilate brain change is drained when we create barriers or resist needed changes in patterns of behavior. Optimal brain performance necessitates a maximal quantity of mental energy. The capacity to sustain mental energy requires a flexible mindset in times of uncertainty, a clear structured approach to managing ambiguity, the required skills, necessary resources, applicable knowledge, well thought through goals, and a commitment to learn, succeed, fall short, learn from mistakes and succeed again.

The brain tends to operate within an established set of mental patterns focusing on what is already known as true, and in doing so will discount new information that is in sharp opposition or lacking consistency to existing patterns of thinking.

The brain's ability to be impervious and resistant to new information blocks, misstates, twists, squanders, exhausts, and contaminates new thinking. Substantive shifts in thinking occur from the perception of opportunity and curiosity while clearly defining the true cost of changing or not changing one's behavioral patterns.

Be prepared for the brain's aha moments. Not knowing is the brain's greatest teacher. Allowing yourself to be surprised at life's surprises is like being on a carnival ride. The brain likes to be explainable and predictable, safe, and to keep on happening just the way we perceive it should be. The belief that we can create a new future is so extraordinary that most of the time we can't bring ourselves to see it for what it is—accepting the opportunity and consequences it would take to actually change our thinking. Behavioral change is simply a matter of trial and correction day-in-day-out. Nothing is certain in life while change continuously challenges our mental capacity.

My hope is that *Good Brain Bad Brain Your Brain* will influence you to consider working on behavioral changes that will influence a new future you. My wish is that you start to think outside your traditional box and practice these nuggets of brain droppings. The process of new thinking will change your brain's neuropathways forever. You can't control the weather, politics, the economy or others yet you can learn to manage your thinking and how you apply that new thought in a more conscious way to your life and satisfaction.

In the process of retraining your brain you will be granted some deeper truth about yourself and your seat in the world. Changing one's script in life is a transformational learning experience. But learning about "what" and "how" you think is a double-edged sword, opening the mind to new possibility and irreversible changes. Knowledge of yourself will influence your idea of self and the world, yet in the pursuit of mental transformation the practices in this book may lead you down the path less traveled. In the process, you may face self-doubt, relapse in behavior, and alienate people you felt were friends. Regardless of what happens I guarantee you will understand who you are which is a sign of progress. In the words of Daryl Conner author of Managing At The Speed of Change, "Nature designed each of us to move through life at a unique pace that will allow us to absorb the major changes we face in the best way possible." Like physical fitness, you can't store or rush the process of transformation. You will only be able to achieve optimal brain performance by understanding how your life circumstances affect your behavior. Brain change can be distilled down to a series of attempts that allow you to adjust to world circumstances, the unknown, uninvited, and the unintended glitches encountered in living ones life. The road to brain transformation is riddled with potholes, detours, unintentional deviations from what is correct, right and true. The messy business of thinking brings to light contradiction, conflicting choices, and resistance. There is no compass for this journey, you will get lost and side tracked along the way but the road to new thinking, health and wellness is worth the time and effort, pain and healing.

17

Your Brain Plan

Coach Conner's Final Words

Many of my clients have one specific request, "tell me what I should do "exactly"?"

I wrestled with this desired "want" for several reasons. Each brain is engineered differently in how we learn, think and communicate or manage daily stress. Then there are environmental circumstances, which have been home grown through previous exposure to people, places and situations, and let's not forget our inherited genetics and patterns of behavior acquired since birth, which influence everything our brains do. My job is not to tell you what to do but rather deepen your learning experience, facilitate that learning experience, and help foster self-awareness. The process of learning consists of the novice brain and the experienced brain, which creates the foundation for your brain's thought process. It is up to you to find the answer, develop a plan and create the strategies for growth and transformation. Good Brain, Bad Brain, Your Brain, gives you the understanding, knowledge and know how to move forward. It is my responsibility as a health and wellness coach to insist that you must acquire this learning for yourself. Telling you what to do "exactly" denies your uniqueness and doesn't help you build confidence in your own ability. The notion of "trial and correction" will provide the mind and body the understanding necessary to develop a conscious mind, then it can be said you have learned the actions, patterns of behavior, and mental attitude needed to change your life circumstances.

The process of thinking is like learning to drive a car. To get your license you had to attend driver's education where you were exposed to educational movies and discussion on safe driving habits and driving regulations. Then you had to practice driving and after that you had to pass a multiple-choice test and take a practical exam with a driving instructor demonstrating your driving skills. Now think back to those first driving lessons, let's face it all that mental preparation didn't really condition your mind or body for the state of preparedness needed to actually drive a car on the road with other cars. Initially you had to over-think every action you took, while trying to recall all the rules of the road. And no one warned you about the potholes, detours, extreme weather conditions, blind spots inside and outside your vehicle and worse, the other drivers. After several close encounters, small fender benders, parking and speeding violations and lots and lots of experience you became a fairly proficient driver. Every new situation opened your mind to "what" is needed to happen and "how" to process each unforeseen encounter. The conscious brain must be present and in the moment to be effective at anything. The brain's competencies are learned the old fashion way through the progressive process of thinking, experiencing, and being. Brain change happens within the mind, allowing concepts, ideas, judgment, and inferences to take hold. The process of thought allows the brain to immediately form fresh neurological connections creating the mindset for new thinking. When the brain is energized through learning and experiences it absorbs and assimilates all that new information. These brain connections are not random but rather a compilation of billions of thought bytes that have been analyzed, scrutinized, identified and categorized within your brain's neuro-pathways. When you decide to change how you and your brain operate what you are trying to do is renegotiate with your brain's hardwired, habitual preferences in behavior. The law of neuroplasticity has shown that with practice we can retrain our brain to imagine a new mind and body blueprint with the choices we make allowing us to minimize future stressors while subsequently growing a new smarter brain. The good news is the brain makes physical changes based on the repetitiveness of our behaviors and experiences in life. The bad news is the brain makes physical changes based on these same repetitive behaviors and experiences. Think about it. The brain actually wires itself and forms brain connections based on what you do repeatedly in your life, whether it is binging on your favorite TV series or sugar fix, sipping a power drink, ordering a grande latte at Starbucks, pouring a glass of wine to unwind after work, smoking cigarettes, taking a prescription to calm down or burning a joint to take the edge off. Whether you call them good or bad habits, healthy or addictions, they become wired into your brain's neuro-pathways.

The idea of neuroplasticity basically means that the brain is not fixed in its anatomical functionality or structure but rather moldable and adaptable. David Perlmutter M.D. a neuroscientist said "Neuroplasticity provides us with a brain that can adapt not only to changes inflicted by damage but allows adaptation to any and all experiences and changes we encounter." In other words, you can be addicted to almost anything because addictive behaviors involve neuroplastic changes in your brain brought on by regular conditioning to a substance or experience whether your talking exercise, shopping, drugs, digital devices, pornography and more.

So if we go back to my driving school example, the knowledge acquired in driving school without actual experience is merely intellectualizing the process of driving and the experience of driving without the knowledge gotten in drivers education is driving under the influence of ignorance. Retraining the brain is an internal change that requires closing the gap between old unnecessary patterns of thinking in light of newer more effective life-brain strategies. All that said here's my best generic take on a brain plan. It all starts with how we think about life.

THE PLAN

CREATE A VISION
Find and define your purpose. This will allow you to articulate and create a compelling vision for your new future and provide you a clear sense of what matters most. When facing habitual behavioral change it is only natural for the brain to instinctively preserve the status quo. Your vision will become the compass, map, and inspiration towards moving forward into the transition state of change allowing your mind to reflect on what you most deeply value. Identify:

- Strengths and Weaknesses
- Past Successes and Learnings
- Challenges and Corrections
- Motivators and Barriers

AWARENESS
Focus on your personal lifescape, which includes everything that affects your behaviors. Become a conscious competent aware of those automatic, unconscious patterns of behavior rooted in the brain's operating system of the neuro-pathways. This will allow you to kick to the curb all mementos that could lessen successful brain change. Take a comprehensive inventory of existing unconscious automatic habits (positive and negative) that take a toll on your mental and physical energy, performance, health and happiness. For example:

. Food consumption
Give your brain a wake-up call by keeping a food journal. This is the ultimate learning tool. Consume high quality calories.
70% Fruits and Veggies (1 fruit, 3 vegetable servings)
20% Protein
10% Fat

. Alcohol
     One drink Friday & Saturday

. Smoking
     Lose the habit

. Junk and fast food
     Lose the habit or minimize the consumption of food products that use sugar, bleached flour, and salt.

. Energy drinks and soda
     Lose the habit. Stop drinking sodas and using products made with artificial sweeteners. Drink water throughout the day. You can use a squeeze of lemon or lime.

. Coffee
     If your caffeine sensitive drink herbal tea. Otherwise you can have approximately 2 cups of java by day.

. Sleep and recovery
     7.5+ to 9 hours of quality sleep by day. Research suggests that when individuals get fewer than six hours of sleep at night, they have lower overall blood flow in the brain, which translates into craving issues and poor decision-making. Over time sleep deprivation causes individuals to be unrealistically and optimistic which tends to lead to risky behaviors.

. Artificial light from computers, cells, tables and other technological devices.
     Turn these devices off in the evening. Artificial light disturbs sleep patterns.

. Exercise
     Cardiovascular training 3-7 days a week 20 minutes to 1 hour

Muscular (strength or endurance) Training 2-3 days a week

. Relationships
No drama or stressful relationships (human, animal, or substance). Life is too short, just move on.

. Mindset – optimistic or pessimistic thinking.
Focus on your physical and emotional health as a transformational discipline. Learn to reframe your circumstances in a positive light. Highly specific routines can manage energy and sustained performance. Start thinking 3 [+] feelings to 1 [-] feeling. Encourage your friends and family to do the same.

SMART Goals
When designing brain changes the most effective and inspirational goals are those describing the actions that stir behavioral change. Your goals need to be **S**pecific, **M**easureable, **A**ction Oriented, **R**ealistic, and **T**imely. When thinking through the behaviors necessary to achieve SMART behavioral goals develop intentions that connect to your vision. It is important to know what you want but it is a brain imperative to know how you're going to get there.

. When thinking through each goal acknowledges to you your level of readiness, confidence, commitment, ability and willingness? You can't change what you haven't acknowledged.

ACTION
This is an opportunity to practice behavioral change. Practicing desired behaviors effects how you act, think and feel creating a positive momentum for change to take hold. Prioritize no more than 2-4 smart goals to work on weekly. Ask yourself:

. What are your health goals? Then ask yourself are you ready then commit to those goals.

. Choose friends and family to support your vision.

. Wake up each day with focused strategies that will ensure you achieve each goal.

. When consuming food at home, eating on the run, or dining out, plan ahead. Remember you can always find a healthy alternative in most restaurants.

. Join online communities, support groups, and spend more time around healthy people.

. Reflect on each moment of each day and celebrate your successes.

. Manage your mental and physical energy like a currency. Energy can be overused and underused. Learn to balance your mind and body energy expenditures with intermittent energy renewal.

. To build mental and physical stamina you must push beyond your comfort zone.

Many psychologists believe these wanted and unwanted patterns of behavior represent all experiences from the moment we open our eyes at birth and by the time we hit our 30's our personality and life story will be completely branded within the brain's neuro-pathways. We have spent literally decades retaining and recalling past experiences, learning behaviors, attaining attitudes which frame our minds and affecting our thoughts, beliefs, reactions, and subconscious perceptions. Think about how drawn out and difficult life would become if you had to overthink brushing your teeth or trying to talk yourself out of what you believe to be true or what if you couldn't draw a conclusion regarding what to eat, what movie to watch, or what friends you should hang with. Life would be a natural disaster. Remind yourself this subconscious programming of the brain operates on autopilot to save the mind and body energy and can be reprogrammed.

To reshape the brain's thinking you must let go of established patterns of behavior held in place by the brain's neuro-emotional filters. Identify those wanted or unwanted patterns of behavior you wish to change only then can you become mentally objective ready to receive new insights and independent thoughts. Our brain's greatest rival is the ability to get the better of our fixed mental conditioning. Retraining the brain starts within the mind. Start by choosing the right mental attitude that supports the right actions generating the desired results. Change is inevitable so take control of your circumstances now before your brain gets pushed off balance and into the hold of resistance. Actively engage change because the need to change doesn't happen simply because it is a good idea. We can pay for brain change up front with new thinking or pay for it on the back end in mind and body healing.

Back to the reason I felt giving you an "exact plan" wouldn't be desirable. Brain change and crisis are co-conspirators. The past has shown us that regardless of how well you plan for habitual change, these challenges reveal the brains emotional state. It comes down to "what" you do and "how" you proceed that matters. Those who are capable of existing in spite of adversity flourish mentally, learning to take advantage of thinking that helps bring about a more resilient brain. There are ways in which our brains attempt to influence behaviors that can justify old thinking or promote a more preferred outcome. The brain always starts by presenting us with an honorable deception as to maintain established thinking denying us a true transformative experience. The brain seeking substantive change and transformation must be open to seeing a point of view otherwise not considered possible. To acquire new thinking that enhances your quality of life, you must be ready, able and willing to embrace the growing burden of brain change without tumbling into a pool of dysfunctional behavior. With the knowledge that our brain can learn to under-

stand and manage what in the past seemed unthinkable, new behaviors can then take root. The decision to change your thinking
is not merely an opportunity to dramatically change your life,
it represents a declaration, an opportunity and responsibility to
live a more effective healthier life through the application of new
thinking. I once read that the notion of true mastery of any skill
requires the patience and dedication of a serious student. Your
plan comes down to choosing the options that will provide you
the life you desire.

References and Further Reading

CHAPTER 1

Daniel Amen, MD, Use Your Brain to Change Your Age, Three Rivers Press, 2012.

Daryl R. Conner, Managing at the Speed of Change, Villard Books, a division of Random House, Inc., 1994.

Suniya S. Luthar, Dante Cicchetti, Bronwyn Becker, The Construct of Resilience: A Critical Evaluation and Guidelines for Future Work, May 31, 2007.

Dante Cicchetti and W. John Curtis, Multilevel perspectives on pathways to resilient functioning, Cambridge University Press, Development and Psychopathology/Volume 19/Issue 03/ Summer 2007 pp. 627-629.

Sutcliffe, K.M. & Vogus, T.J. (2003). Organizing for Resilience. In Cameron, K., Dutton, J.E., & Quinn, R.E. (Eds.), Positive Organizational Scholarship. San Francisco: Berrett-Koehler. Chapter 7 pp.: 94-110

Garmezy N. Resilience in children's adaptation to negative life events and stressed environments. Pediatrics. Sep; 1991; 20:459-466

Masten, A. S. Resilience in individual development: Successful adaptation despite risk and adversity. In M. C. Wang & E. W. Gorden (Eds.), Educational resilience in inner city America 1994;(pp. 3-25). Hillsdale, NJ: Erlbaum.

George R. Uhl, MD, PhD; Robert W. Grow, MS, The Burden of Complex Genetics in Brain Disorders, Arch Gen Psychiatry. 2004; 61 (3): 223-229.doi: 10.1001/archpsyc.61.3.223

CHAPTER 2

Antonio Damasio, Self Comes to Mind: Consturcting the Conscious Brain, 1010.

Antonio Damasio, Descartes' Error: Emotion, Reason, and the Human Brain, Putnum; revised Penguin edition, 2005.

Antonio Damasio, The Feeling of What Happens: Body and Emotion in the Making of Consciousness, Harcourt, 1999. Nelson Cowan, Working Memory Capacity. Hove, East Sussex, UK: Psychology Press, 2005.

Nelson Cowan, Attention and Memory: An integrated framework. Oxford Psychology Series (no.26). New York: Oxford University Press, 1997.

Nelson Cowan, M. L. Courage, The development of memory in infancy and childhood. Hove, U.K.: Psychology Press, 2009.

The Franklin Institute, Resources for Science Learning. webteam@www.fi.edu

Justin Rhodes, PhD and researcher at Beckman Institute. www.beckman.illinois.edu/news/Rhodes040910

Brenda Patoine, Move Your Feet, Grow New Neurons? Exercise –Induced Neurogenesis Shown in Humans, May 1, 2007. www.dana.org/printerfriendly.aspx?id=7374

Dan Hurley, Can You Build a (Better Brain?), A new working-memory game has revived the tantalizing notion that people can make themselves smarter. The New York Times, April 22, 2012.

John Lehrer, How We Decide, 2009; HOUGHTON MIFFLIN HARCOURT.

Daniel B. Levinson, Jonathan Smallwood, Richard J. Davidson, The Persistence of Thought, Evidence for a Role of Working Memory in the Maintenance of Task-Unrelated Thinking, April 16, 2012.

Barbara Strauch, author of The Secret Life of the GROWN-UP BRAIN, 2010.

Hara Estroff Marano, Psychology Today, What Is Good Brain Food? October 01,2003.

D.L. Korol and P. E. Gold, Abstract on Glucose, memory and aging. The American Journal of Clinical Nutrition, 1998.

Harris R. Lieberman, Military Nutrition Division, US Army Research Institute of Environmental Medicine (USARIEM), NATICK, MA OL760-5007, USA, Appetite, Volume 40, Issue 3, June 01, 2003, Pages 245-254.

Nelson Cowan, The Development of Memory in Childhood 1997. Chapter 7, Pages 163-166.

Alan D. Baddeley, Human Memory: Theory ad Practice, 1997.

Gary Taubes, Do We Really Know What Makes Us Healthy? New York Times Magazine, September 16, 2007, 52.

Michael Pollan, In Defense of Food, New York Penguin Press, 2008.

Michael Pollan, Unhappy Meal, New York Time Magazine, January 2007, 38.

Nicholas Bakalar, Study Critiques Antioxidant Supplements, New York Times, April 29, 2008, Sec. F.

The National Institute of Health (NIH) http://intranet.ninds.nih.gov/employee/neurosciencenews/ne urosciencenews.2006.htm

Maesako M, Uemura K, Kubota M, Kuzuya A, Sasaki K, Hayashida N, Asada-Utsugi M, Watanabe K, Uemura M, Kihara T, Takahashi R, Shimohama S, Kinoshita A., , Exercise Is More Effective than Diet Control in Preventing High Fat Diet-induced B-Amyloid Deposition and Memory Deficit in Amyloid Precursor Protein Transgenic Mice. J Biol Chem. 2012 Jun 29;287(27): 23024-33. Epub 2012 May 4.

Barbara L. Fredrickson, Ph.D. Positivity, Three River Press, January 27th, 2009.

Avi Zenilman, Slate Magazine, The Rules of Distraction, November 18, 2005.

Porter Anderson, CNN.com/Career, Study: Multitasking is counterproductive, December 6, 2001.

Claudia Wallis, The Multitasking Generation, Time Magazine, Friday March 24, 2006, Professor David Meyer is quoted in Time Magazine's March 27th, 2006 issue.

Randall Kaplan, Carol Greenwood, Gordon Winocur, and Thomas MS Wolever.The American Journal of Clinical Nutrition, Dietary protein, carbohydrate, and fat enhance memory performance in the healthy elderly 1'2'3', November 2001, vol. 74 no. 5 687-693.

deRegnier RA, Nelson CA, Thomas KM, Wewerka S, Georgieff MK. Neurophysiologic evaluation of auditory recognition memory in healthy newborn infants and infants of diabetic mothers. J Pediatric. 2000; 137:777-84.

Lisman JE, Grace AA. The hippocampal-VTA Loop: controlling the entry of information into long-term memory. Neuron. 2005; 46: 703-13.

USDA, Agricultural Research Service, James A. Joseph USDA-ARS Human Nutrition Research Center on Aging at Tufts University. Nutrition and Brain Function, August issue of Agricultural Research Magazine.

Kretchmer N. Beard JL, Carlson S. The role of nutrition in the development of normal cognition. American Journal of Clinical Nutrition. 1996; 63:S997-1001.

Burden MJ, Westerland AJ, Armony-Sivan R, Nelson CA, Jacobson study of attention and recognition memory in infants with iron-deficiency anemia. Pediatrics. 2007; 120:e336-45. JAMA, August 12, 2009; abstracts at jama.ama-assn.org/cgi/content/abstract/302/6/627. Alzheimer's Association, www.alz.org.

Focus on Healthy Aging, Mount Sinai School of Medicine. Maintaining Health and Vitality in Middle Age and Beyond. Volume 10G-R.

Nutrition Action, September 2012. David Schardt, Brainmakers, Can popping pills preserves memory?

Charles Fernyhough, Pieces of Light, 2012.

CHAPTER 3

Locke, E. A. & Lathan, P.P. 2002 Building a practically useful theory of goal setting and task motivation: A 35 year odyssey. American Psychologist, 57(9), 705-717.

John C. Briggs and F. David Peat, Looking Glass Universe: The Emerging Science of Wholeness, Simon and Schuster, June 1986.

Edward de Bono, de Bono's, Thinking Course, 1994 by MICA Management Resources, published by Facts On File, Inc.

Alan O. Ross, Personality: Theories and Processes, July 3, 1992, Harper Perennial, a division of Harper Collins Publishers.

Daniel G. Amen, M.D., Use Your Brain to Change Your Age, April 4th, 2012, Three River Press.

Daryl R. Conner, Managing at the Speed of Change, January 19th, 1993, Villard Books, NYC, Random House, Inc.

Barbara Zoltan, MA, OTR/L, Vision, Perception, Cognition: A Manual for the Evaluation and Treatment of the Adult with Acquired Brain Injury, Fourth Edition, January 18th, 2007

Richard Paul and Linda Elder, Critical Thinking: Tools for Taking Charge of Your Professional and Personal Life, Financial Times-Prentice Hall, An imprint of Pearson Education, 2002.

Antonio Damasio is David Dornsife Professor Neuroscience, and Psychology, Self Comes to Mind, 2010, Random House, Inc.

Shelley Carson, Ph.D., Your Creative Brain, Jossey-Bass, 2010.

Johnmarshall Reeve, Understanding Motivation and Emotions, John Wiley & Sons, Inc., 2009.

Gollwitzer, P.M., & Oettigen, G., History of the concept of motivation. In J. Smelser & P.B. Baltes (Eds.). International Encyclopedia of the Social and Behavioral Science (pp.10100-10112). Oxford, U.K.: Elsevier Science Ltd., 2001.

Norbert Schwarz, SCIENCE WARCH, Self-Reports, How the Questions Shape the Answers, February 1999, American Psychologist.

Bernard Weiner, An Attributional Theory of Achievement Motivation and Emotion, Psychological Review, 1985, Vol. 92, No.4, 548-573, by the American Psychological Association, Inc.

Lewis, F.M. and Daltroy, L. H., How Casual Explanations Influence Health Behavior. Attribution Theory. Jossey-Bass Publishers Inc. 1990. Bodenhausen, G. V., & Morales, J. R. (2013). Social cognition and perception. In I. Weiner (Ed.), Handbook of psychology (2nd ed., Vol. 5, pp. 225-246).

Hoboken, NJ: Wiley.Bodnhausen, G. V., Kang, S. K., & Peery, D. (2012). Social categorization and the perception of social groups. In S. T. Fiske & C. N. Macrae (Eds.), SAGE handbook of social cognition (pp. 311-329). Los Angeles, CA: Sage.

Gawronski, B., & Bodenhausen, G. V. (2012). Self-insight from a dual-process perspective. In S. Vazire & T. D. Wilson (Eds.), *Handbook of self-knowledge* (pp. 22-38). New York: Guilford Press

CHAPTER 4

See Lester Coch and John R. P. French, Jr., Overcoming Resistance to Change, Human Relations, Vol. 1, No. 4, 1948, p. 512.

Daryl R. Conner, Managing at the Speed of Change, Villard Books, 1994, a division of Random House, Inc., Chpt. 8, p. 125.

Thomas R. Harvey and Elizabeth A. Broyles, Resistance to Change: A Guide to Harnessing Its Positive Power, Rowman & Littlefield Publishers, Inc., June 16, 2010.

Brien Palmer, Making Change Work: Practical Tools for Overcoming Human Resistance, ASQ Quality Press, 2004.

Weiten, W. & Lloyd, M.A. Psychology Applied to Modern Life (9th ed.). 2008, Wadsworth Cengage Learning.

Zeidner, M. & Endler, N.S. (editors) Handbook of Coping: Theory, Research, Applications, 1996, New York: John Wiley.

R. S. Lazarus & S. Folkman, *Stress, Appraisal, and Coping,* Springer Publishing Company, March 15, 1984.

Goleman, Daniel, *Emotional Intelligence: Why It Can Matter More Than IQ,* Bantam Books, Sep 27, 2005.

Dale H. Emery, Resistance As A Resource, Cutter IT Journal Vol. 14 No. 10, October 2001.

Bridges, William. *Managing Transitions.* Reading, Mass: Addison-Wesley, 1991.

Elgin, Suzette Haden. *BusinessSpeak.* New York: McGraw-Hill, 1995.

Weinberg, Gerald M. *Quality Software Management, Volume 2: First-Order Measurement.* New York: Dorset House Publishing, 1993.

Susan M. Heathfield, How to Reduce Resistance to Change, http://humanresources.about.com/od/resistancetochange/a/how-to-reduce-resistance-to-change.htm.

CHAPTER 5

Malcolm Gladwell, Outliers: The Story of Success, Little, Brown and Company, November 2008.

Eknath Easwaran, Take Your Time: How to Find Patience, Peace, and Meaning, Nilgiri Press, 1994-2006 by The Blue Mountain Center of Meditation.

Jonah Lehrer, Patience, http://scienceblogs.com/cortex/2010/05/06/patience/ Effective Mind Control, What is Patience? http://www.effective-mind-control.com/what-is-patience.html

Dr. Joe Dispenza, Breaking the Habits of Being Yourself, Hay House, Inc., 2012.

Gordon Linvingston, M.D., Too Soon Old, Too Late Smart, DaCapo Lifelong, 2004.

AMA, American Management Association, Secrets of Multitasking: Slow Down to Speed UP., http://www.amanet.org/training/articles/Secrets-of-Multitasking-Slow-Down-to-Speed-Up.aspx

Eknath Easwaran, Take Your Time: The Wisdom of Slowing Down, The Blue Mountain Center of Meditation, 2006.

Ferris Jabr, Scientific America, Why Your Brain Needs More Down Time, October 15, 2013, http://www.scientificamerican.com/article/mental-downtime/

Mind Tools, How to be Patient, Staying Calm Under Pressure, http://www.mindtools.com/pages/article/newTCS_78.htm.

KR Consulting, Kristin Robertson, Patience is a Leadership Virtue, June 2004, http://www.krconsulting.com/patience-is-a-leadership-virtue/

Davi Johnson Thornton, Brain Culture, A British Cataloging-in-Publication record, 2011.

Susan Fiske and Shelly E. Taylor, Social Cognition: From Brain to Culture, Sage Publication, Ltd., January 15, 2013.

P.M.H. Atwater, Future Memory, Hampton Roads Publishing Company, Inc. 2013

CHAPTER 6

Rogers, R. & Monsell, S. (1995). The costs of a predictable switch between simple cognitive tasks. *Journal of Experimental Psychology: General,* 124, 207-231.

Rubinstein, Joshua S.; Meyer, David E.; Evans, Jeffrey E. (2001). Executive Control of Cognitive Processes in Task Switching. *Journal of Experimental Psychology: Human Perception and Performance,* 27(4), 763-797.

Multitasking May Not Mean Higher Productivity. (2009). Talk of the Nation, National Public Radio. Found online at http://www.npr.org/templates/story/story.php?storyId=11233444 9

American Psychological Association. (2006). Multitasking: Switching costs. Found online at http://apa.org/research/action/multitask.aspx

Herbert Alexander Simon, Professor and Nobel Prize Winner Scholarly Articles for Monet/Lazarus and Technological Stress Journal of Further Education Vol.14, Issue 3, Sept. 1990

Richard S. Lazarus, PhD. Professor of Psychology at University of California Berkley, Stress, Appraisal and Coping, Effect of Voluntary Control on Performance Response Under Stress, 1984 New York: Springer

Arnetz, Wihol, and Muter
Technological Stress: Psychophysiological Symptoms in Modern Offices, Journal of Psychosomatic Research, Vol 43, Number 1, July 1997.

Lazarus and Muter, Assessing and Managing Technostress, Psychological Stress and Coping Processes 1984, McGraw Hill.

Arnetz Techno-Stress. Psycho-physiological consequences of poor man-machine interface. 1993 Case Study.

CHAPTER 7

Catherine Steiner-Adair, EdD with Teresa H. Barker, The Big Disconnect, Harper Collins Publishers, 2013.

Henry Jenkins, Convergence Culture, New York Press, 2006.

Dana Boyd, It's Complicated, Yale University Press, 2014.

Clara Shih, The Facebook Era, Pearson Education Inc., 2011.

Winifred Gallagher, RAPT, Attention and the Focused Life, The Penguin Press, 2009.

Fowler JH, Dawes CT, Christakis NA (2009) Model of genetic variation in human social networks. Proc Natl Acad Sci USA 106:1720-1724.

Moody J (2001) Race, school integration, and friendship segregation in America. Am J Sociol 107:679-716.

Jackson MO, Rogers BW (2007) Meeting strangers and friends of friends: How random are social networks? Am Econ Rev 97:890-915.

Olson JM Vernon PA, Harris JA, Jang KL (2001) The heritability of attitudes: A study of Twins. J Personality Soc Psychol 80:845-860

Katie Pinholster, LPC, CRC – Pinholster Family Counseling www.pinholsterfamilycounseling.com

CHAPTER 8

R. A. Hegele, Premature atherosclerosis associated with monogenic insulin resistance, *Circulation* 103 (2001): 2225-2229.

Frances Sizer and Eleanor *Whitney, Nutrition Concepts and Controversies,* 9th addition

David A. Kessler, MD, The end of overeating.

Hegele RA, Reue K. Hoofbeats, zebras, and insights into insulin resistance. J Clin Invest 2009; 119:249-251. (PMID: 19244606).

Ley SH, Harris SB, Mamakeesick M, Noon T, Fiddler E, Gittelsohn J, Wolever TM, Connelly PW, Hegele RA , Zinman B, Hanley AJ. Metabolic syndrome and its components as predictors of incident type 2 diabetes mellitus in an Aboriginal community. *CMAJ*, 2009; 1

Joy T, Kennedy BA, Al-Attar S, Rutt BK, Hegele RA . Predicting abdominal adipose tissue among women with familial partial lipodystrophy. Metabolism 2009; 58:828-834.

David A. Kessler, MD, *The end of overeating.* Rodale Books 2009.

Dr. Phil McGraw, *The Ultimate Weight Solution.* The Free Press and colophon 2003.

Barbara Rolls, PhD., *The Volumetrics Eating Plan,* Harper Collins Publishers 2005.

John Cloud, Why Exercise Won't Make You Thin, *Time* August 17, 2009. Laurette, Antoine Bechara, Alain Daher, and Adam Drewnowski, *Obesity Prevention: The Role of Brain and Society on Individual Behavior.*

Ball, K. and Crawford, D. "An Investigation of Psychological, social, and environmental Correlates of Obesity and Weight Gain in Young Women." *International Journal of Obesity*, 30, NO. 8 (2006): 1240-49.

Norman, D.A. and Shallice, T. "Attention to Action: Willed and Automatic Control of Behavior." In Gazzaniga, M.S. Cognitive Neuroscience: A READER. OXFORD: BLACKWELL, 2000.

David A. Levitsky, Ph.D., *Malnutrition, Environment, and Behavior: New Perspectives* 1978.

Terry Nicholetti Garrison and David A. Levitsky, Ph.D., *Fed-Up: A Woman's Guide to Freedom From Diet/Weight Prison* 1993.

Jacqueline H. Beckley MBA, M. Michele Foley, Elizabeth J. Topp and Jack C. Huang, *Accelerating New Food Product Design* and Development (Institute of Food Technologists Series) 2007.

Howard R. Moskowitz Ph.D., Jacqueline H. Beckley MBA, Anna V. A. Resurreccion Ph.D., *Sensory and Consumer Research in Food Product Design and Development* (Institute of Food Technologists Series) 2006.

Kelly Brownell Ph.D. and Katherine Battle Horgen, *Food Fight: The Inside Story of the Food Industry, America's Obesity Crisis, and What We Can Do About It 2004.*

Kelly Brownell Ph.D., *The Learn Program For Weight Management 2000.*

Elaine A. Blechman Ph.D. and Kelly Brownell Ph.D., *Behavioral Medicine and Women: A Comprehensive Handbook 1999.*

G. Terence Wilson Ph.D., Cyril M. Frank, and Kelly D. Brownell, Ph.D., Annual Review of Behavior Therapy, Volume 9: Theory and Practice 1984.

Ronald A. Ruden, *The Craving Brain: A Bold New Approach to Breaking Free from *Drug Addiction, *Overeating, *Alcoholism, and *Gambling 2000.*

Ronald A. Ruden, *The Craving Brain: The BioBalance Approach to Controlling Addictions 1997.*

Nina Frusztajer Marquis and Judith J. Wurtman, *The Serotonin Power Diet: Use Your Brain's Natural Chemistry to Cut Cravings, Curb Emotional Overeating, and Lose Weight 2006.*

Paul Rivas, MD and E. A. Tremblay, *Turn Off The Hunger Switch Naturally: The Revolutionary New Program That Resets Your Brains Chemistry for Real Weight Loss without Cravings and Hunger 2003.*

Shiffrin, R. M. and Schneider, W. *Controlling and Automatic Human Information Processing: II: Perceptual Learning, Automatic Attending and A General Theory,* Psychological Review, 84, No. 2 (1977): 127-90.

Mike Dow, PsyD, Interview with clinical director of therapeutic and behavioral services at The Body Well Integrative medical center in Los Angeles and host and psychotherapist of the TLC series Freaky Eaters. Bottom Line , September 15, 2011, page 9 and 10. On the web: www.BottomLine Secrets.com.

Jeffrey Luger, TIME September 13, 2010, Pages 45 – 49.

Dr. Phillip C. McGraw's, Give Yourself a Mental Makeover, OPRAH.com, September 2010, page 78-79.

Rahael Moeller Gorman, ADDICTED TO FOOD? Eating Well, 79 Nutritional Report. March 2011.

Howard Fields-UCSF School of Medicine, M.D., Ph.D. Professor of *Neurology* Director, Wheeler Center for the Neurobiology of Addiction Principal Investigator. Interview in David Keller's book The end of overeating.

Saul Shiffman, Addiction, Volume 95, Issue 8s2, pages 171-175, August 2000.

Marcia Levin Pelchat, Food Cravings in Young and Elderly Adults, Appetite, Volume 28, Issue 2, February 1997, Pages 103-113, ELSEVIER.

Hormes, J. & Rozin, P. (2009). Premenstrual chocolate craving. What happens after menopause? Appetite, 53 (2), 256-259.

Rory Evans, Craving Control, Allure, September 1, 2008. PMS and the work of Marcia Pelchat.

Dr. Stephen Gullo, psychologist, professor and researcher at Columbia University Medical Center. Thin Tastes Better, October 7, 1998, Dell Health, and The Thin Commandments January 1, 2005

Carl C. Pfeiffer, PhD., MD, Mental and Elemental Nutrients, Keats, CT, 1975, p.24

P. Willner, D. Benton, E. Brown, S. Cheeta, G. Davies, J. Morgan, M. Morgan, Depression increases "craving" for sweet rewards in animal and human models of depression and craving. Psychopharmacology, 136(3): 272-83, Apr 1998.

Dr. Jennie MacDiarmid, Marion M. Hetherington, Mood modulation by food: an exploration of affect and cravings in 'chocolate addicts'. British Journal of Clinical Psychology, 34(pt.1): 129-38, Feb 1997.

Marion M. Hetherington, Food Cravings and Addictions, Aug 2001.

James L. Groff, Sareen S. Gropper, Sara M. Hunt. Advanced Nutrition and Human Metabolism, West Publishing Company, M, 1995, 373.

Dallas Clouatre, PhD., Getting Lean with Anti-Fat Nutrients, Pax Publishing, CA 1993, p.22. and Dr. Clouatre's Corner, Glykon Technologies Group, LLC.

Harold H. Sandstead, MD and Nancy W. Alcock, PhD. Zinc: an essential and unheralded nutrient. Journal of Laboratory and Clinical Medicine, 197: 130(2):116-118. As cited in Clinical Pearls 1997 pg. 271.

Benard Jenson, PhD., The Chemistry of Man, B. Jensen Publisher, 1983, deficiencies linked to specific cravings and some food recommendations. >Neuroscience Lett. 79: 138, 1987

Marcovitch, S., Jacques, S., Boseovski, J. J., & Zelazo, P. D. (2008). Self-reflection and the cognitive control of behavior: Implications for learning. Mind, Brain, and Education, 2, 136-141.

Cunningham, W. A., & Zelazo, P. D. (2010). The development of iterative reprocessing: Implications for affect and its regulation. In P. D. Zelazo, M. Chandler, & E. A. Crone (Eds.). Developmental social cognitive neuroscience (pp. 81-98). Mahwah, NJ: Lawrence Erlbaum Associates

Silvia A. Bunge and Jonathan D. Wallis, Neuroscience of Rule-Guided Behavior, Oct 5,2007

Pamela Peeke, MD, The Hunger Fix: The Three –Stages Detox and Recovery Plan for Overeating and Food Addiction, September 18, 2012, Dr. Pamela Peeke's 10 Weight-prevention tips, Discovery Health. http://health.howstuffworks.com/wellness/diet-fitness/weight-loss/10-toxic-weight-prevention-tips.htm

CHAPTER 9

Frances Sizer and Eleanor Whitney, Nutrition Concepts and Controversies, ninth edition.

L. Kathleen Mahan and Sylvia Escott-Stump, Krause's Food, Nutrition & Diet Therapy.

National Institute on Alcohol Abuse and Alcoholism (NIAAA):

Neuroscience: Pathways to Alcohol Dependence Part II--Neuroadaptation, Risk, and Recovery, Vol. 31, No. 4, 2008

Neuroscience: Pathways to Alcohol Dependence Part 1--Overview of the Neurobiology of Dependence, Vol. 31, No. 3, 2008

Alcohol and Other Drugs, Vol. 31, No. 2, 2008

Systems Biology: The Solution to Understanding Alcohol-Induced Disorders?, Vol. 31, No.1, 2008

Alcohol Metabolism Part II: A Key to Unlocking Alcohol's Effects, Vol. 30, No.1, 2007

Alcohol Metabolism Part I: Mechanisms of Action, Vol. 29, No. 4, 2006

Alcohol and Tobacco: An Update, Vol. 29, No. 3, 2006

National Epidemiologic Survey on Alcohol and Related Conditions: Selected Findings, Vol. 29, No. 2, 2006

Health Services Research, Vol. 29, No.1, 2006

Focus on Young Adult Drinking, Vol. 28, No. 4, 2004/2005

Screening and Brief Intervention, Part II-A Focus on Specific Settings, Vol. 28, No. 2, 2004/2005

Screening and Brief Intervention, Part 1-An Overview, Vol. 28, No. 1, 2004/2005

Alcoholic Liver Disease, Part II-Mechanisms of Injury, Vol. 27, No. 4, 2003

Alcoholic Liver Disease, Part 1-An Overview, Vol. 27, No. 3, 2003

Alcoholic Brain Disease, Vol. 27, No. 2, 2003

Epidemiology in Alcohol Research, Vo. 27, No. 1, 2003

Women and Alcohol: An Update, Vol. 26, No. 4, 2002

Genetic Technology in Alcohol Research, Vol. 26, No. 3, 2002

Alcohol and Comorbid Mental Health Disorders, Vol., 26, No. 2, 2002

Preventing Alcohol-Related Problems, Vol. 26, No. 1, 2002

Alcohol-Related Birth Defects: An Update, Vol. 25, No. 3, 2001

Alcohol and Violence, Vol. 25, No. 1, 2001

Life Science Editorial Services:

>   Alcoholism: Clinical & Experimental Research

>   Drug & Alcohol Dependence

>   Alcohol & Alcoholism

>   Alcohol

>   Journal of Studies on Alcohol

>   American Journal of Drug & Alcohol Abuse

>   Addiction

>   American Journal of Epidemiology

>   International Journal of Epidemiology

Alcohol Research Group, Public Health Institute:

>   National Institute on Alcohol Abuse and Alcoholism

>   National Institute on Drug Abuse

>   National Institutes of Health

>   National Institutes on Mental Health http://www.nmh.nih.gov

>   National Clearinghouse for Alcohol and Drug Information (NCAD) http://ncadi.samhsa.gov/

>   National Association of State Alcohol and Drug Abuse Directors (NASADAD) http://www.nasadad.org/

>   Substance Abuse & Mental Health Services Administration http://www.samhsa.gov/

>   College Drinking Prevention, NIAAA http://www.collegedrinkingprevention.gov/

>   Drug Policy Alliance http://www.drugpolicy.org/homepage.cfm 281

CHAPTER 10

Robert W. Levenson, Unraveling Emotional Mysteries, Observer Vol. 27, No. 1 January 2014.

Rob Stein, Do We Choose Our Friends Because They Share Our Genes? NPR, July 14, 2014.

Loyola University Health System, Science Daily, What falling in love does to your heart and brain. February 6, 2014.

Daniel Amen, The Brain in Love: 12 Lessons to Enhance Your Love Life. Three Rivers, 2009.

Different cognitive processes underlie human mate choices and mate preferences – PNAS. "Proceedings of the National Academy of Sciences. Web. 06 November 2009. http://www.pnas.org/content/104/38/15011. Abstract

The Science of Romance: Why We Love-TIME." Breaking News, Analysis, Politics, Blogs, News Photos, Video, Tech Reviews – TIME.co, Web. 06 November. 2009. http://www.time.com/time/magazine/article/0,99171,1704672,00. html.

True Love and Chemistry: Exploring Myth and Reality. "ENotAlone

Relationship advice and articles. Web. 06 November. 09 http://www.enotalone.com/articles/2946.html.

Brenda Schaeffer. Is it Love or Is It Addiction? Hazelden, 2009. Print.

Helen. Romantic Love: An fMRI Study of a Neural Mechanism for Mate Choice. N. Page print.

Martin E. P. Seligman, Ph.D., Authentic Happiness, Free Press 2002.

Alan O. Ross, Personality: Theories and Processes, Harper Collins College Outline, Pg. 193-194 Harpers Collins Publishing, Inc. 1992.

Winifred Gallager, RAPT, Attention and the Focused Life, The Penguin Press, 2009.

Gordon Livingston, M.D., Too Soon Old, Too Late Smart, Da Capo Press Books, 2004.

CHAPTER 11

Martin E. P. Seligman, PhD., Authentic Happiness 2002.

Gordon Livingston, M.D., Too Soon Old, Too Late Smart, Da Capo Press Books, 2004.

Carol S. Dweck, PhD., Mindset 2006.

Daryl R. Conner, Managing at the Speed of Change 1993.

Dr. Phil McGraw, The Ultimate Weight Solution 2003.

Barlow, D. 1988, *Anxiety and Its Disorders: The Nature and Treatment of Anxiety and Panic.* New York: Guilford.

Lazarus, R. S., and S. Folkman, 1984, *Stress, Appraisal, and Coping:* New York: Springer Publishing.

Jessop DS, Harbuz, MS, Lightman SL. CRH in chronic inflammatory stress. Peptides. 2001 May; 22(5):803-7. Review.

Michael Olpin and Margie Hessen, *Stress Management for Life: A Research-Based Experiential Approach,* 2006.

CHAPTER 12

Christopher G. Langton a computer scientist and author of *Artificial Life: An Overview (Complex Adaptive System),* 1997.

Steven Johnson author of *Where Good Ideas Come From,* 2010.

Daryl R. Conner author of *Managing at the Speed of Change,* 1994. Workbook, *Fundamentals of the MOC Methodology,* 1995.

Ned Herrmann, *The Creative Brain,* 1988.

David C. McClelland, Boston University, *Human Motivation,* 1987.

Carol Dweck, C., Self theories: The role of motivation, personality and development, 1999, Random House.

Carol Dweck, The New Psychology of Success, 2003, Random House.

Howard Gardner, Frames of mind: The theory of multiple intelligences. 1983. Basic Books.

Howard Gardner, Multiple intelligences: New horizons. 2006, Basic Books.

Richard J. Heurer Jr., Phychology of Intelligence Analysis, 2007, Pherson Associates.

Ronald Kotulak, Inside the Brain: Revolutionary Discoveries of How the Mind Works. 1997, Andrews McMeel Publishing.

Arthur L. Costa and Bena Kallick, Learning and leading with Habits of Mind: 16 Essential Characteristics for Success, 2009, Association for Supervision and Curriculum Development.

CHAPTER 13

Immanuel Kant, Paul Guyer, and Allen W. Wood, Critique of Pure Reason, Cambridge University Press, February 28, 1999.

Stephen R. Covey, The 7 habits of Highly Effective People: Powerful Lessons in Personal Change by Stephen R. Covey, Rosetta Books LLC, New York, November 9, 2004.

Joe Dispenza DR. Breaking The Habits of Being Yourself: How to Lose Your Mind and Create a New One, Hay House, Inc., February 15, 2013.

Hebb, D.O., The Organization of Behavior: A Neuropsychological Theory. (Mahwah, NJ: Lawrence Erlbaum Associates, Inc., 2002)

Dr. Joe Dispenza, Breaking the Habit of Being Yourself, Hay House, Inc., 2012.

Daniel G. Amen, Use Your Brain to Change Your Age, 2012.

Szegedy-Maszak, Marianne, "Mysteries of the Mind: Your unconscious is making your everyday decisions."U.S. News & World Report, February 28, 2005.

Church, Dawson, Ph.D., The Genie in Your Genes: Epigenetic Medicine and the New Biology of Intention, Santa Roasa, CA: Elite Books, 2007.

Yue, G., and K.J. Cole, "Strength increases from the motor program: comparison of training with maximal voluntary and imagined muscle contractions," Journal of Neurophysiology, vol. 67(5): 1114-1123 (1992)

Wallace, B. Alan, Ph.D., The Attention Revolution: Unlocking the Power of the Focused Mind, Boston: Wisdom Publication, Inc., 2006.

CHAPTER 14

Daryl R, Conner, *Managing at the Speed of Change,* 1992.

Steven Johnson, *Where Good Ideas Come From,* 2010.

Jim Loehr and Tony Schwartz, *The Power of Full Engagement,* 2003.

Barbara Strauch, *The Secret Life of the Grown-up Brain,* 2010.

Daniel Kripke, Psychologist and researcher, Journal of Sleep Research and supported by the National Institute of Health, www.wiley.com/bw/journal.asp?ref=0962-1105

Richard R. Bootzin, John F. Kihlstrom, and Daniel L. Schacter, *Sleep and Cognition,* July 1990.

Gerard A. Kerkhof and Hans Van Dongen, *Human Sleep and Cognition, Part II, Volume 190: Clinical and Applied Research (Progress in Brain Research),* May 29th, 2011.

Timothy H. Monk, *Sleep, Sleepiness, and Performance (Wiley Series in Human Performance and Cognition,* December 1991.

YOO, SS, ET AL, *A Deficit in The Ability to Form New Human Memories Without Sleep,* Natural Neuroscience, 10 NO.3, March 2007: 38592.

Marshall, L and J Born, *The Contribution of Sleep to Hippocampus Dependent Memory Consolidation,* Trends in Cognition in Science, 11 NO. 10, October 2007: 442.50.

Jim Loehr and Tony Schwartz, The Power of Full Engagement, 2003.

Marine Corps University Web, an article written by the military concerning sleep deprivation.

WEB search
Marine Corp web site:
http://www.mcu.usmc.mil/tbsnew/pages/infantry/human factor/page4.htm.-Article on sleep deprivation.

Sara Ledoux, article on The Effects of Sleep Deprivation on Brain and Behavior, January 2008.

http://www.articlebase.com/health-articles/the-amazing-link-between-sleep-and-memory-1328356.html#ixzz1DmYaOAZq

Michael J. Gleb, *How to Think Like Leonardo De Vinci,* 1998.

Sigmund Freud, *The Interpretation of Dreams,* 1900.

Sarah Van Boven, *BEAUTY BY NUMBERS, Sleep,* Allure/ January 2008.

Vladimir Nabokov, *Speak, Memory,* 1966. University of California San Diego, Study of brain activity and sleep deprivation.

Carol Honore, *In Praise of Slowness,* 2004.

National Sleep Foundation 2007.

Gerard A Kerkhof and Hans Van Dongen, Human Sleep and Cognition, Volume 185: Basic Research (Progress in Brain Research), January 21, 2011.

CHAPTER 15

Edward F. Pace-Schott, Mark Solms, Mark Blagrove, Steven Garnad, Sleep and Dreaming: Scientific Advances and Reconsiderations, Cambridge University Press, 2003.

Penelope A. Lewis, The Secret World of Sleep: The Surprising Science of the Mind at Rest, Palgrave Macmillian 2013.

Martha David, Elizabeth Robbins Eshelman, Matthew McKay, The Relaxation & Stress Reduction Workbook, New Harbinger Publications, Inc., 2008.

Karyn Repinski, SHAPE Magazine, April 2014, p. 154.

National Sleep Foundation. 2003 Sleep in America Poll. Online: www.sleepfoundation.org

Gregg D. Jacobs, Say Good Night to Insomnia: The Six-Week, Drug-Free Program Developed at Harvard Medical School, Henry Holt and Company 1998.

Your Guide to Healthy Sleep. U.S. Department of Health and Human Services, National Institutes of Health, National Heart, Lung, and Blood Institute. NIH Publication No. 06-5271. November 2005. Online: www.NHLBI.NIH.gov/health/public/sleep/healthy_sleep.pdf

American Insomnia Association
www.americaninsomniaassociation.org

American Sleep Apnea Association www.sleepapnea.org

Narcolepsy Network, Inc. www.narcolepsynetwork.org

National Sleep Foundation www.sleepfoundation.org

Restless Legs Syndrome Foundation www.rls.org

American Board of Sleep Medicine www.absm.org

Geriatric Mental Health Foundation www.gmhfonline.org˝©

www.ingramcontent.com/pod-product-compliance
Lightning Source LLC
Chambersburg PA
CBHW060844280326
41934CB00007B/919